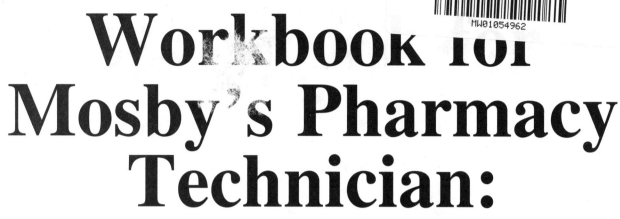

# Workbook for Mosby's Pharmacy Technician:
## Principles and Practice, 2nd edition

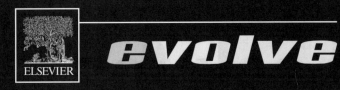

**∴** *To access your Instructor Resources, visit:*

# http://evolve/elsevier.com/Hopper/

Evolve Student Learning Resources for *Hopper: Workbook for Mosby's Pharmacy Technician: Principles and Practice* offer the following features:

## Instructor Resources

- **Chapter Weblinks**
  These links offer you the opportunity to check your understanding and execute the workbook web-based research assignments, plus expand your knowledge base and stay current with this ever-changing industry.

- **English/Spanish Audio Glossary**
  This audio glossary helps reinforce terminology reviewed in the Terms and Definitions section and helps you with difficult pronunciations.

- **Anatomy Animations**
  These animations provide a visual learning tool that covers not only basic anatomy, but body functions as well.

The Latest Evolution in Learning.

Evolve provides online access to free learning resources and activities designed specifically for the textbook you are using in your class. The resources will provide you with information that enhances the material covered in the book and much more.

Visit the Web address listed below to start your learning evolution today!

# Workbook for Mosby's Pharmacy Technician:
## Principles and Practice

## SECOND EDITION

Teresa Hopper, BS, CPhT

Instructor of Pharmacy Technology
San Joaquin Valley College
Rancho Cordova, California

Karen Snipe, CPhT, AS, BA, MAEd

Pharmacy Technician Program Coordinator
Trident Technical College
Charleston, South Carolina

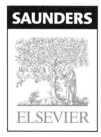

SAUNDERS

ELSEVIER

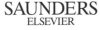

SAUNDERS
ELSEVIER

An Imprint of Elsevier

11830 Westline Industrial Drive
St. Louis, Missouri 63146

WORKBOOK FOR MOSBY'S PHARMACY TECHNICIAN:          ISBN 13 978-1-4160-3782-8
PRINCIPLES AND PRACTICE, 2nd edition               ISBN 10 1-4160-3782-9
**Copyright © 2007, 2004, by Saunders, an imprint of Elsevier, Inc.**

**All rights reserved.** No part of this publication may be reproduced or transmitted in any form or by any means, electronic or mechanical, including photocopy, recording, or any information storage and retrieval system, without permission in writing from the publisher.
Although for mechanical reasons all pages of this publication are perforated, only those page imprinted with an Elsevier, Inc. copyright notice are intended for removal.
Permissions may be sought directly from Elsevier's Health Sciences Rights Department in Philadelphia, PA, USA: phone: (+1) 215 239 3804, fax: (+1) 215 239 3805, e-mail: healthpermissions@elsevier.com. You may also complete your request on-line via the Elsevier homepage (http://www.elsevier.com), by selecting "Customer Support" and then "Obtaining Permissions".

**Notice**

Neither the Publisher nor the Authors assume any responsibility for any loss or injury and/or damage to persons or property arising out of or related to any use of the material contained in this book. It is the responsibility of the treating practitioner, relying on independent expertise and knowledge of the patient, to determine the best treatment and method of application for the patient.

The Publisher

ISBN 13: 978-1-4160-3782-8
ISBN 10: 1-4160-3782-9

Publishing Director: Andrew Allen
Executive Editor: Loren Wilson
Developmental Editor: Lynda Huenefeld
Publishing Services Manager: Julie Eddy
Senior Project Manager: Rich Barber
Designer: Andrea Lutes

Printed in the United States

Last digit is the print number:  9  8  7  6  5  4

Working together to grow
libraries in developing countries

www.elsevier.com | www.bookaid.org | www.sabre.org

ELSEVIER    BOOK AID International    Sabre Foundation

# Preface

This student workbook is designed to help you master the information and skills presented in your textbook: *Mosby's Pharmacy Technician: Principles and Practice*, 2nd edition. The various types of exercises will challenge your knowledge, help further reinforce key content, and allow you to gauge your understanding of the subject matter you have studied in the respective chapters of your textbook. The following list explains the types of exercises contained in this student workbook:

- *Terms and Definitions:* Terms and definitions are listed, preceded by a letter. You are to read each statement following the list, and write in the letter that represents the correct response. This exercise helps you recall the many terms that are introduced to you in each chapter. Your textbook conveniently lists this information at the beginning of each chapter. If you find you are not sure of any of your responses, you an easily turn to the appropriate chapter to refresh your memory.
- *Fill in the Blanks:* Complete each statement by filling in the blanks. This exercise gives you the opportunity to specifically apply the vocabulary you have learned within the context of pharmacy.
- *True or False:* Test your knowledge of the validity of the statements. If you think a statement is true, write a "T" in the blank preceding the statement; if you believe it is a false statement, write in an "F." Completing these exercises helps you immediately to recognize content of which you are unsure. You can then review and strengthen your understanding of the material by rereading that particular section in your textbook.
- *Multiple Choice:* You are to select the one best answer to complete the numbered questions by circling the letter preceding the answer you have selected. This is the type of question in which your first response is usually the correct reply. If you are not sure, then you can easily review the subject in question.
- *Body System Practice:* Each chapter devoted to a body system features an illustration of the system with its organs numbered. You are asked to identify the organs contained in the body system. This visual exercise helps further reinforce your knowledge of anatomy. Questions in these chapters test you on the anatomy and physiology of the system, diseases and conditions that may occur within this system, and the medications prescribed to treat such illnesses.
- *Matching:* These exercises provide you with essential practice in matching controlled substance drug schedules with given drug names. Ease of recognition is essential in your chosen profession. If you are not sure of some of your responses, you can then refer back to your textbook for further study.
- *Lab Sheets:* Lab Sheets for specific chapters will help you master such skills as gram staining, interpreting abbreviations, performing conversions and calculations, and loading patient medication drawers. These exercises offer you opportunities for hands-on reinforcements of what you have learned in your textbook.
- *Conversion and Calculation:* These questions require you to convert measurements, thereby applying what you have learned.
- *Research Activities:* You are asked to use the Internet as a research tool to assist you in locating essential information. Featured websites address such topics as the scope of practice for pharmacy technicians and where to find information on controlled substances and recalls.
- *Critical Thinking:* This exercise tests your accumulated knowledge of each chapter by giving you scenarios to solve. You are asked to draw upon your knowledge of pharmacy and direct it to specific situations. This is a good test of your understanding of key concepts. If any of these questions stump you, refer back to your textbook for further study, or ask your instructor for clarification.

# Contents

# 1 History of Medicine and Pharmacy

## TERMS AND DEFINITIONS

Select the correct term from the following list and write the corresponding letter in the blank next to the statement.

A. Apothecary

B. Dogma

C. Inpatient pharmacy

D. Outpatient pharmacy

E. Pharmacist

F. Pharmacy clerk

G. Pharmacy technician

H. Shaman

I. Protocol

J. Clinical pharmacist

_____ 1. Code of beliefs based on tradition rather than fact

_____ 2. Community pharmacies or pharmacies in outpatient hospital settings

_____ 3. Person who dispenses drugs and counsels patients

_____ 4. Person who assists the pharmacist at the front counter of the pharmacy

_____ 5. Latin term for pharmacist

_____ 6. A pharmacy in a hospital or institutional setting

_____ 7. A spiritual person in a tribe who cares for the spiritual, medicinal, and physical health of the tribe

_____ 8. Person who assists the pharmacist by filling prescriptions and performing other nondispensing tasks

_____ 9. Set of standards written by a hospital or insurance company for patient treatment

_____ 10. Pharmacist who monitors patient medications in inpatient and some retail settings

## IMPORTANT PEOPLE WHO HAVE INFLUENCED THE HISTORY OF MEDICINE

Select the correct name from the following list and write the corresponding letter in the blank next to the description.

A. Aristotle

B. Aesculapius

C. Galen

D. Hippocrates

E. Roger Bacon

F. Gregor Mendel

G. Paracelsus

_____ 1. Scientist and monk, known as the father of genetics

_____ 2. God of medicine in Greek mythology

_____ 3. Greek physician and scientist

_____ 4. Greek philosopher, considered the father of medicine

_____ 5. English scientist responsible for scientific methods

_____ 6. Greek physician who proved that blood flowed through arteries

_____ 7. Swiss physician, philosopher, and scientist

Copyright © 2007 Elsevier, Inc. All rights reserved.

## MULTIPLE CHOICE

Complete each question by circling the best answer.

1. The placebo effect
   A. Works from the outside of the body to the inside
   B. Works by placing the drug over the area to be treated
   C. Works because the patient strongly believes it will work
   D. Works only after midnight

2. Trephining is
   A. A radical treatment that lasted for hundreds of years
   B. A term used to describe menstrual bleeding
   C. Draining of the poisonous blood from the sick person
   D. An incision into the skull to create an exit portal for disease

3. In early America, doctors were
   A. Responsible for diagnosing conditions
   B. Responsible for preparing the necessary remedy
   C. The first druggists
   D. All of the above

4. The division between physicians and pharmacists began after the
   A. Korean War
   B. Civil War
   C. Vietnam War
   D. Cold War

5. Cisterns were
   A. Jars used to store medicinal ingredients
   B. A special knife used for removing cysts
   C. A folk name for girls in the same family
   D. A recipe book for ailments

6. Early remedies in American history included
   A. Cinchona bark (quinine) to treat malaria
   B. Mercury to treat syphilis
   C. Opium and alcohol to treat pain
   D. All of the above

7. The first pharmacy technicians were
   A. Military personnel
   B. High school graduates
   C. Family members of the pharmacist
   D. Certified pharmacy technicians (CPhTs)

8. In early years the typical pharmacist was a person who
   A. Wore a white jacket
   B. Worked the soda machine
   C. Packaged up the medications
   D. All of the above

9. In some states, today's typical pharmacy technician
   A. Is required to do an array of tasks
   B. Is required to be educated and an OJT
   C. Is a family member of the pharmacist
   D. Both A and B

10. How can technicians gain the trust of the patients they serve?
    A. Education
    B. Training
    C. Good communication skills
    D. All of the above

11. The concept that doctors act only for the good of the patient and keep confidential what they learn about their patients reflects the
    A. Galenic Oath
    B. Corpus Hippocratum
    C. Hippocratic Oath
    D. De Materia Medica

12. The effectiveness of the opium and alcohol mixture was surpassed only by its
    A. Addictiveness
    B. Availability
    C. Adverse effects
    D. All of the above

## FILL IN THE BLANK

1. Technicians help the pharmacists by preparing _____ and _____.

2. Name four duties of technicians in a hospital setting:

   A. _____

   B. _____

   C. _____

   D. _____

3. Name two areas of pharmacy a pharmacist can specialize in:

   A. _____

   B. _____

4. The most important thing a patient can develop for a technician is _____.

2

                    Copyright © 2007 Elsevier, Inc. All rights reserved.

## SHORT ANSWER

1. State the Hippocratic Oath. _____

_____

_____

_____

2. What is the difference between an opioid and opium? _____

_____

_____

_____

3. What does the term *dogma* mean? _____

_____

_____

_____

## RESEARCH ACTIVITY

1. Access the website *www.ptcb.org* and investigate the duties outlined for pharmacy technicians.

2. Access the website *www.pharmacy.wsu.edu/history*. List five facts from the account on the history of pharmacy.

## CRITICAL THINKING

1. One of the most important aspects of a pharmacy technician's job is to gain the trust of the pharmacist. How would you, as a new technician on the job, go about gaining the trust of the pharmacist?

2. What changes have you seen in pharmacy as a consumer over the years?

3. How have medicinal treatments changed from ancient beliefs to present-day practices? Start with the shamans and conclude with twenty-first century medicine.

Copyright © 2007 Elsevier, Inc. All rights reserved.

# 2 Law and Ethics of Pharmacy

## LAWS AND DEFINITIONS

Select the correct law from the following list and write the corresponding letter in the blank next to the statement.

A. 1906 = Federal Food and Drug Act

B. 1914 = Harrison Narcotic Act

C. 1938 = Food, Drug and Cosmetic Act

D. 1951 = Durham-Humphrey Amendment

E. 1962 = Kefauver-Harris Amendment

F. 1970 = Comprehensive Drug Abuse and Prevention and Control Act

G. 1983 = Orphan Drug Act

H. 1987 = Prescription Drug Marketing Act

I. 1990 = Anabolic Steroids Control Act

J. 1990 = Omnibus Budget Reconciliation Act

K. 1996 = The Health Insurance Portability and Accountability Act

L. 2005 = Combat Meth Act 2005

_____ 1. Required drug companies to include directions for use for the consumer in package inserts on drugs; required the marking "Warning: May be habit forming" for all narcotics

_____ 2. Attempted to ensure the safety and effectiveness of all new drugs introduced to the market

_____ 3. Enacted to stop the sale of inaccurately labeled drugs

_____ 4. Required the label "Caution: Federal law restricts this drug to use by or on the order of a licensed veterinarian" for certain drugs

_____ 5. States that a pharmacist must counsel all patients who receive new prescriptions at the time of purchase

_____ 6. Created an agency with the sole purpose of enforcing the laws governing narcotics and the requirements for their distribution

_____ 7. Enacted because of excessive opium addiction across the United States

_____ 8. Deals with a person's right to continuance of health insurance even when the individual changes employers

_____ 9. Helped stiffen regulations dealing with the abuse of anabolic steroids and their misuse by athletes

_____ 10. Made the initial distinction between a legend drug and over-the-counter drugs; required legend drugs to carry the label "Caution: Federal law prohibits dispensing without a prescription"

_____ 11. Allowed drug companies to bypass the lengthy time requirements for testing of a new drug, and the costs that accompany them, to provide medications to persons who have a rare disease

_____ 12. Addresses all areas of the manufacturing, enforcement of laws, and sale of methamphetamines made from pseudoephedrine

Copyright © 2007 Elsevier, Inc. All rights reserved.

## TRUE OR FALSE

Write T or F next to each statement.

_____ 1. The FDA regulates the manufacture and safe-guarding of medications.

_____ 2. Thalidomide, a drug prescribed to help people sleep, caused children to be born without limbs and with severe defects; this was a widespread problem throughout the United States.

_____ 3. The Orphan Drug Act was passed for diseases that affect fewer than 200,000 persons in the United States.

_____ 4. All patients must be given information on the drugs they are taking, such as the drug's name, when to take it, how long to take it, and any side effects or possible interactions.

_____ 5. Technicians will not be held liable if they do not know all the new and upcoming changes relating to HIPAA.

_____ 6. Not all controlled substances are addictive.

_____ 7. The FDA and DEA were both created under the Department of Justice.

_____ 8. HIPAA is a federal act that protects patients' health.

_____ 9. The strictest law (federal versus state) is the one employees of the pharmacy must follow.

_____ 10. Not all prescribers must be registered with the DEA to write prescriptions for narcotics.

## MULTIPLE CHOICE

Complete the question by circling the best answer.

1. Who has the authority to decide under what schedule a drug should be placed?
   A. RPh
   B. FDA
   C. Attorney general
   D. DEA

2. A C-III drug can be refilled
   A. 0 times
   B. 2 times
   C. 5 times
   D. 6 times

3. A prescription for a C-IV drug expires after
   A. 14 days
   B. 3 months
   C. 6 months
   D. 12 months

4. A drug monograph is
   A. A picture of the drug
   B. Literature on the drug
   C. Literature on the manufacturer
   D. A price list for the drug

5. Phone order prescriptions can be received by
   A. Pharmacy clerks
   B. Pharmacy interns
   C. Pharmacy technicians
   D. Pharmacists

6. Prescriptions for controlled substances are designated with a "C" that must be
   A. In red in the lower right corner of the prescription
   B. In black in the lower right corner of the prescription
   C. In red in the lower left corner of the prescription

   D. In black in the lower left corner of the prescription

7. Which of the following numbers could be the DEA number for Dr. Green?
   A. AB5527835
   B. AG5387255
   C. AB5387255
   D. BG5378255

8. Which medication does not require a childproof cap?
   A. Amoxicillin chewable tablets
   B. Nitrostat SL tablets
   C. Mycelex troche
   D. Amoxicillin suspension

9. The highest level of manufacturer's recall, which indicates products that could cause serious harm or fatalities, is a
   A. Class 1 recall
   B. Class 2 recall
   C. Class 3 recall
   D. Class 4 recall

10. A tort is
    A. A small fruit pie
    B. The amount of force used to inject a needle
    C. A type of instrument used in compounding
    D. Causing injury to a person intentionally or because of negligence

11. For a pharmacy to obtain schedule II controlled substances from a distributor, which DEA form must be filled out?
    A. 122
    B. 222
    C. 324
    D. 306

  Copyright © 2007 Elsevier, Inc. All rights reserved.

12. Which of the following controlled substance schedule drugs can be obtained OTC?
   A. C-II
   B. C-III
   C. C-IV
   D. C-V

13. Invoices for C-II drugs must be kept for _____ years.
   A. 2
   B. 4
   C. 5
   D. 7

## FILL IN THE BLANK

1. Which reference text do physicians use to access drug information? _____

2. Recommended dosing is usually specified by _____ and _____.

3. Which government agency allows consumers and health care professionals to report discrepancies or adverse reactions to medications? _____

4. What two pieces of information are needed on a prescription label?
   _____ and _____

5. The pharmacy technician's clear responsibility on many levels is the _____.

6. _____ are morals in the workplace.

7. Taking _____ orders for prescriptions is not within the pharmacy technician's scope of practice.

## MATCHING

Match the controlled substance designations with the correct drug.

_____ 1. C-II          A. Vicodin

_____ 2. C-III         B. LSD

_____ 3. C-V           C. Demerol

_____ 4. C-I           D. Valium

_____ 5. C-IV          E. Lomotil

## SHORT ANSWER

1. Explain the various components of the DEA#:

_____

_____

_____

   A. What do the letters represent? _____

_____

_____

   B. How do you verify that a DEA# is authentic? _____

_____

_____

2. What did the Poison Prevention Act of 1970 address and create? _____

_____

_____

_____

Copyright © 2007 Elsevier, Inc. All rights reserved.

## RESEARCH ACTIVITY

1. Access the website *www.fda.gov*. Find information on controlled substances and recent drug recalls.

2. Use the website *www.fda.gov/fdac/features/2001/501_drug.html* to find information on prescription drug use and abuse.

## CRITICAL THINKING

1. If you could add one more law to the existing laws addressing the abuse of prescription medications, what would it be?

2. Marijuana has been the subject of debate lately for possible medicinal use in patients with cancer and AIDS. Into which controlled substance schedule would you put it if it were approved for such use?

3. Someone presents a C-II prescription in the pharmacy 31 days after it was written. Knowing that C-II drugs must be filled within 30 days of the original date written, how would you tell the patient that this prescription cannot be filled?

8

Copyright © 2007 Elsevier, Inc. All rights reserved.

# 3 Pharmacy Settings for Technicians

## TRUE OR FALSE

Write T or F next to each statement.

_____ 1. Each of the 50 states in the United States has standardized the qualifications and job descriptions for pharmacy technicians.

_____ 2. Each state has its own board of pharmacy that is overseen by the NABP.

_____ 3. Pharmacy technicians perform nonjudgmental tasks, such as counseling patients.

_____ 4. _Inpatient pharmacy_ refers to pharmacy for patients who are in the hospital for an overnight stay or longer.

_____ 5. All documentation in the inpatient pharmacy is based on a 24-hour cycle.

_____ 6. Preparing unit-dose medications is an outpatient technician duty.

_____ 7. It is more important to be fast and concise than to be correct and complete.

_____ 8. Outpatient pharmacy is one of the most difficult tasks in pharmacy.

_____ 9. In-home health care technicians process medications usually on a weekly or monthly basis.

_____ 10. All pharmacy technician jobs are performed in a pharmacy.

## PHARMACY TECHNICIAN JOB OPPORTUNITIES

Select the correct job from the following list and write the corresponding letter in the blank next to the description.

A. Inventory technician

B. Robot filler

C. Chemo technician

D. Clinical technician

E. Insurance technician

F. Technician recruiter

G. Technician trainer

H. PBM operator

I. Computer support technician

J. Poison Control Call Center operator

_____ 1. Trains newly hired technicians in computer programs and other skills relevant to their pharmacy

_____ 2. Interprets orders and prepares all chemotherapeutic agents

_____ 3. Supports personnel with automated medication dispensing systems

_____ 4. Knows Medicare, Blue Cross, and other insurance companies' guidelines

_____ 5. Recruits technicians into their outpatient or temporary agencies

_____ 6. Orders and bills all stock

_____ 7. Screens incoming calls and transfers calls to 911 operator or pharmacist; authorized to take the call if it concerns a minor issue

_____ 8. Assists the pharmacist with tracking patient's medications

_____ 9. Is trained to load mechanical equipment and keep it running smoothly

_____ 10. Helps customers over the phone

Copyright © 2007 Elsevier, Inc. All rights reserved.

## MULTIPLE CHOICE

Complete the question by circling the best answer.

1. The board of pharmacy
   A. Registers pharmacists and technicians
   B. Provides a way for consumers to report complaints, problems, or illegal pharmacy actions
   C. Reviews and updates current pharmacy rules and regulations
   D. All of the above

2. The term *nonjudgmental* means that technicians can perform
   A. Tasks that require little or no thought
   B. Tasks in a pharmacy setting that must be checked and approved by a pharmacist
   C. Tasks that require interpretation of scientific studies
   D. Tasks that are unethical

3. Pharmacy technicians are *not* required to keep which of the following hospital units stocked?
   A. ICU
   B. OR
   C. ATM
   D. CCU

4. Medications need to be repackaged in unit-dose because
   A. Medication is not available in unit-dose.
   B. This is a hospital cost savings.
   C. A and B
   D. None of the above

5. Which job is *not* a common inpatient technician responsibility?
   A. Preparing insurance billing
   B. IV technician
   C. Chemo technician
   D. Anticoagulant technician

6. Which of the following is *not* a typical outpatient technician responsibility?
   A. Taking new prescriptions over the phone
   B. Refilling prescriptions
   C. Answering questions about various insurance plans
   D. Ordering stock

7. In the home health care setting, which of the following is *not* a typical pharmacy technician responsibility?

   A. Processing medication prescriptions
   B. Filling prescriptions for walk-in patients
   C. Filling blister packs
   D. Providing services for home health nurses

8. In the mail order or E-pharmacy setting, which of the following is *not* a common technician responsibility?
   A. Refilling prescriptions
   B. Processing new prescriptions
   C. Using computers
   D. Preparing IV meds

9. The national certification examination is given
   A. 50 times a year
   B. Four times a year
   C. Only for hospital technicians
   D. Three times a year

10. Which of the following is *not* a goal of the Pharmacy Technician Certification Board?
    A. To ensure that technicians work equally and for the same pay as pharmacists
    B. To provide greater patient care and service
    C. To create a minimum standard of knowledge
    D. To help employers determine the technician's knowledge base

11. Stat orders are to be delivered within _____ minutes to the nursing stations requesting them.
    A. 60
    B. 30
    C. 15
    D. 5

12. Which of the following is *not* an aspect of inpatient pharmacy?
    A. Preparing parenterals
    B. Preparing hyperalimentation
    C. Preparing chemotherapy
    D. Preparing patient billing

13. Which of the following is *not* an eligibility requirement for taking the PTCB exam?
    A. High school diploma
    B. Graduate of a pharmacy technician program
    C. No convictions for a drug-related felony
    D. GED

## FILL IN THE BLANK

1. Name three high-volume duties in an outpatient pharmacy:

   A. _____

   B. _____

   C. _____

   Copyright © 2007 Elsevier, Inc. All rights reserved.

2. Home health clinics provide _____ _____ _____ and are taken care of by _____ in the _____ home.

3. Certified technicians use the designation _____ after their name.

4. _____ hours of CE are required yearly to retain certification.

5. Name five opportunities for the educated technician that are "nontraditional" duties:

A. _____

B. _____

C. _____

D. _____

E. _____

6. What types of pharmacy knowledge are tested in the PTCB certification exam?

A. _____

B. _____

C. _____

D. _____

E. _____

## RESEARCH ACTIVITIES

1. Call or visit a local retail pharmacy and a hospital pharmacy. Ask the lead technician or the pharmacist in charge the following questions.
   A. What qualifications do you require for technicians in your pharmacy?
   B. What duties do your technicians perform?
   C. Do you require certification?

2. Access the website *http://pharmacytechnician.org*. Read what this organization is doing for pharmacy technicians and find out about the requirements for membership.

3. Access your state board of pharmacy on the Internet. (First access *www.nabp.net* and look for your state board of pharmacy listing.) What does the Pharmacy Practice Act say about technicians?

4. Review the classified ads in a local newspaper and study any job description listed for pharmacy technicians.

5. What types of activities or benefits do the ASHP and the APhA offer technicians?

**11**

Copyright © 2007 Elsevier, Inc. All rights reserved.

1. You have been asked to advise someone interested in becoming a pharmacy technician. How would you advise this person?

2. What is your definition of professionalism with regard to pharmacy technicians?

3. As a new technician on the job, you believe that you have not been given enough training for your new job duties. How long do you think new employees should receive training when starting a new job?

Copyright © 2007 Elsevier, Inc. All rights reserved.

# 4 Conversions and Calculations Used by Pharmacy Technicians

## TERMS AND DEFINITIONS

Select the correct term from the following list and write the corresponding letter in the blank next to the statement.

A. Alligation

B. Apothecary system

C. Avoirdupois system

D. International time

E. Metric system

F. Volume

G. Household

_____ 1. A system of measurement based on multiples of 10

_____ 2. A system of measurement used in pharmacy

_____ 3. A method of determining the needed amounts of two different concentrations to prepare a needed concentration

_____ 4. A 24-hour method of keeping time with no distinguishing between AM and PM

_____ 5. The amount of liquid enclosed in a container

_____ 6. A system of measurement used to determine weight

_____ 7. A system of measurement commonly used for weight, volume, and length in the United States

## TRUE OR FALSE

Write T or F next to each statement.

_____ 1. The ability to manipulate conversions is a required competency of pharmacy technicians.

_____ 2. Not all transcriptions and calculations need to be checked by a pharmacist.

_____ 3. The metric system is used throughout pharmacy because it is the easiest to remember.

_____ 4. All measurements used in pharmacy must be converted to the household system for the patient.

_____ 5. About 90% of all pharmacy calculations are ratio-proportion equations.

_____ 6. The technician should show the parent of a pediatric patient how to measure the correct dosage.

_____ 7. Most IV piggyback solutions are given over 30 to 60 minutes.

_____ 8. One of the most common errors made in pharmacy is placing a zero in front of a decimal.

_____ 9. When conversion is done using the household system, the decimal must be moved either to the right or to the left.

_____ 10. Roman numerals and Arabic numbers are both used in pharmacies.

_____ 11. International time is also known as military time.

_____ 12. It is not important for the technician to double check the calculations because the pharmacist will check them.

Copyright © 2007 Elsevier, Inc. All rights reserved.

Complete each question by circling the best answer.

1. The cost of 100 g of hydrocortisone powder is $36.00. What would be the cost of 12 g?
   - A. $5.42
   - B. $4.32
   - C. $10.60
   - D. $8.94

2. A 125-pound patient weighs how many kilograms?
   - A. 0.125
   - B. 125,000
   - C. 56.82
   - D. 275

3. Convert 1200 mg to grams.
   - A. 12,000 g
   - B. 12 g
   - C. 120 g
   - D. 1.2 g

4. Volume refers to
   - A. Liquids
   - B. Dry ingredients
   - C. Distance
   - D. None of the above

5. The weight of 1 grain is
   - A. 60 mg
   - B. 64 mg
   - C. 65 mg
   - D. All of the above

6. There are 1000 milligrams in 1
   - A. Kilogram
   - B. Gram
   - C. Milligram
   - D. Microgram

7. A patient who weighs 633 kg weighs how many pounds?
   - A. 0.633
   - B. 1392.6
   - C. 287.73
   - D. 28.77

8. 0.005 teaspoon = _____ fluid ounces.
   - A. 3335
   - B. 3.335
   - C. 1.667
   - D. 1667.5

9. A pharmacy wants to increase the price of a product by 35%. How much would an item cost with this markup if its original cost was $6.75?
   - A. $6.95
   - B. $8.21
   - C. $12.50
   - D. $9.11

10. The approximate size of a container for dispensing 120 mL of a liquid medication would be
    - A. 6 oz
    - B. 4 oz
    - C. 8 oz
    - D. 2 oz

11. A physician orders ampicillin 0.5 g PO q6h. The medication available is ampicillin 125 mg/5 mL. What is the quantity of medication to be administered?
    - A. 20 mL
    - B. 2 mL
    - C. 0.2 mL
    - D. 0.02 mL

12. The physician orders atropine 1/150 gr PO bid. The atropine available is 0.4 mg per tablet. The nurse will administer how many tablets per dose? (use 60 mg/gr)
    - A. 0.5
    - B. 0.75
    - C. 1
    - D. 1.5

13. A prescription is written for Pen VK 500 mg tabs PO qid for 10 d. The patient, who has throat cancer and cannot swallow, requests a liquid form. What volume of a 250 mg/5 mL suspension should be dispensed?
    - A. 40 mL
    - B. 400 mL
    - C. 150 mL
    - D. 250 mL

14. A pharmacist dispenses 300 mL of amoxicillin 150 mg/5 mL suspension. The sig is 250 mg PO tid μg. How many days will the prescription last?
    - A. 7 days
    - B. 10 days
    - C. 12 days
    - D. 14 days

15. The doctor's order is for Timoptic ii gtts ou bid. How many drops will the patient get in 12 days?
    - A. 4 drops
    - B. 48 drops
    - C. 69 drops
    - D. 96 drops

16. You receive an order for Kaopectate 15 mL bid prn. One dose equals how many tablespoonfuls?
    - A. 2
    - B. 3
    - C. 1
    - D. Z\x

Copyright © 2007 Elsevier, Inc. All rights reserved.

17. Mylanta and Donnatal are to be combined in a 2:1 ratio. How many milliliters of each are required to make 120 mL of the suspension?
    A. 70 mL/50 mL
    B. 50 mL/70 mL
    C. 80 mL/40 mL
    D. 40 mL/80 mL

18. An IV solution is ordered to run at 3.5 gtts/min. It contains 875 mg in a total of 250 mL. How many milligrams will the patient receive per hour if the set is calibrated to deliver 12 gtts/mL?
    A. 0.16 mg/hr
    B. 16 mg/hr
    C. 61 mg/hr
    D. 610 mg/hr

19. The Roman numeral VLIII is equivalent to
    A. 43
    B. 48
    C. 53
    D. 58

20. Convert 12:14 AM to military time.
    A. 1214
    B. 0214
    C. 0014
    D. 0140

21. The Roman numeral LVIII is equivalent to
    A. 58
    B. 48
    C. 38
    D. 68

22. How many days will the following prescription last?
    Zoloft 100 mg #90
    Sig: 1 PO bid
    A. 55 days
    B. 30 days
    C. 45 days
    D. 90 days

23. A dose is written for 10 mg/kg every 12 hours for 1 day. The adult taking this medication weighs 165 pounds. How much drug will be needed for this order?
    A. 425 mg
    B. 950 mg
    C. 750 mg
    D. 1500 mg

24. How much medication would be needed for the following prescription?
    Prednisone tablets 10 mg
    One qid for 6 days; one tid for 3 days; one bid for 1 day; then stop
    A. 35
    B. 15
    C. 25
    D. 45

25. Using the following DEA formula, what should be the last digit of this DEA number?
    AB461853____
    DEA formula: Add 1st  3rd  5th =
    Add 2 (2nd  4th  6th) = _____
    Total = last digit on the right should be the last digit of the number
    A. 7
    B. 4
    C. 2
    D. 8

26. A dosage of 0.5 g/5 mL is prescribed. You have in stock 150 mg/mL. How many milliliters would be given using the dosage strength on hand?
    A. 2 mL
    B. 5 mL
    C. 3.3 mL
    D. 1.5 mL

27. How many milligrams of bretylium chloride are needed to prepare 3 L of 1:30,000 solution?
    A. 0.1 mg
    B. 1 mg
    C. 10 mg
    D. 100 mg

28. How many liters of a 0.9% normal saline solution can be made from 60 g of NaCl?
    A. 6.67 L
    B. 66.7 L
    C. 667 L
    D. 6667 L

29. If 5 mL of diluent is added to a vial containing 2 g of a drug for injection, resulting in a final volume of 5.8 mL, what is the concentration in milligrams per milliliters of the drug in the reconstituted solution?
    A. 0.3 mg/mL
    B. 345 mg/mL
    C. 444 mg/mL
    D. 2035 mg/mL

30. Which prescription instructions would require 21 tablets to be dispensed?
    A. One tab PO bid for 8 d
    B. One tab ac hs for 4 d
    C. One tab tid for 3 d; one tab bid for 3 d; one qd for 3 d
    D. Three tabs bid for 2 d; two tabs qd for 3 d; one tab qd for 3 d

31. How many grams of potassium permanganate are required to prepare 2 quarts of a 1:750 solution of potassium permanganate?
    A. 0.05 g
    B. 0.13 g
    C. 1.28 g
    D. 13 g

**15**

Copyright © 2007 Elsevier, Inc. All rights reserved.

Chapter **4**  **Conversions and Calculations Used by Pharmacy Technicians**

32. If the dose of a drug is 35 mg/kg/day in six divided doses, how much would be given in each dose to a 38-pound child?
    A. 17.3 mg
    B. 60.4 mg
    C. 101 mg
    D. 604 mg

33. How many grams of yellow mercuric oxide must be added to 30 g of 1% yellow mercuric oxide ointment to prepare a 5% ointment? (Use the alligation method.)
    A. 0.8 g
    B. 1.26 g
    C. 28.9 g
    D. 71.3 g

34. How many capsules, each containing C\, gr of a drug, can be filled completely from a 28 g bottle of the drug?
    A. 24
    B. 32
    C. 313
    D. 431

35. An IV solution containing 20,000 units of heparin in 500 mL of 0.45% NaCl solution is to be infused to provide 1000 units of heparin per hour. How many drops per minute should be infused to deliver the desired dose if the IV set calibrates at 15 gtt/mL?
    A. 0.42 gtt/min
    B. 6 gtt/min
    C. 16 gtt/min
    D. 32 gtt/min

## CONVERSIONS

Convert the following measurements:

1. 8 ounces = _____ mL
2. 90 mL = _____ oz
3. 3 kg = _____ g
4. 2 pints = _____ cups
5. 3.5 = _____ %
6. B\x/ = _____ %
7. Z\c gr = _____ mg
8. 55 lb = _____ kg
9. 125 kg = _____ lb
10. 2500 mL = _____ L
11. 0.15 mg = _____ µg
12. 3600 mL = _____ pts
13. 78 mg = _____ gr
14. Z\c = _____ decimal
15. X\b = _____ decimal

Roman numerals and Arabic numbers

1. XV _____
2. XCIV _____
3. 250 _____
4. 49 _____
5. MDX _____
6. XXXIII _____
7. 125 _____
8. 60 _____
9. IX _____
10. CC _____

## SHORT ANSWER

1. Give the units used in the metric system for the following:

    A. Volume _____

    B. Weight _____

    C. Distance _____

Chapter **4** **Conversions and Calculations Used by Pharmacy Technicians**

Copyright © 2007 Elsevier, Inc. All rights reserved.

2. Give the units used in the household system for the following:

   A. Volume _____

   B. Weight _____

   C. Distance _____

3. Give the units used in the apothecary system for the following:

   A. Liquids _____

   B. Dry weights _____

4. Give the units used in the apothecary system for the following:

   A. Liquids _____

   B. Weights _____

Copyright © 2007 Elsevier, Inc. All rights reserved.

# 5 Dosage Forms, Abbreviations, and Routes of Administration

## TERMS AND DEFINITIONS

Select the correct term from the following list and write the corresponding letter in the blank next to the statement.

A. Absorption

B. Bioavailability

C. Bioequivalence

D. Distribution

E. Excretion

F. Half-life

G. Inhale

H. Instill

I. MDI

J. OTC

K. Parenteral

L. Pharmacokinetics

M. Metabolism

_____ 1. The difference between a drug that is manufactured in a different dosage form or by a different company; includes the rate of absorption, distribution, metabolism, and excretion

_____ 2. The amount of time required for a chemical to be decreased by one half

_____ 3. Metered dose inhaler

_____ 4. The life of the drug, which includes absorption, metabolism, distribution, and excretion

_____ 5. Medication introduced other than by way of the intestines

_____ 6. To place into; instructions used for ophthalmics or otics

_____ 7. The ability of a drug to pass into the bloodstream

_____ 8. The incorporation of a chemical agent across natural barriers within the body

_____ 9. The process of elimination of medicinal agents

_____ 10. To breathe in; directions used for an inhaler

_____ 11. Over-the-counter medications that do not require a prescription

_____ 12. The amount of drug that reaches its intended destination by being absorbed into the bloodstream

_____ 13. The process that breaks down drugs for excretion

## TRUE OR FALSE

Write T or F next to each statement.

_____ 1. To become proficient in the medical profession, a technician must be able to interpret orders correctly.

_____ 2. Much of the terminology used in pharmacy comes from the Latin and Greek languages.

_____ 3. It is not necessary for the pharmacy technician to learn all the dosage forms and abbreviations to decipher a doctor's orders.

_____ 4. The number of errors resulting from doctors' poor handwriting or from transcription of orders is of little concern.

_____ 5. The *dosage form* is the means by which a drug is available to use.

_____ 6. An emulsion is a liquid dosage form.

_____ 7. A troche is a semisolid dosage form.

Copyright © 2007 Elsevier, Inc. All rights reserved.

____ 8. An emulsifier binds oil and water together in a mixture.

____ 9. Enemas typically take longer than 10 hours to work.

____ 10. Semisolid dosage forms are normally meant for topical applications.

____ 11. Gels contain medication in a very viscous liquid that easily penetrates the skin and does not leave a residue.

____ 12. Lozenges are oral tablets that should be swallowed immediately.

____ 13. Doctors frequently use eye solutions to treat ear conditions.

____ 14. A patient's age, gender, genetics, and diet, as well as other chemicals in the body, can influence and alter metabolism.

____ 15. If inhalers are not used properly, medication is swallowed rather than inhaled into the lungs.

## MULTIPLE CHOICE

Complete each question by circling the best answer.

1. The directions for use of a medication are "ii gtts os bid." The route of administration is
   A. Right eye
   B. Left eye
   C. Right ear
   D. Left ear

2. Which of the following is the abbreviation for "before meals"?
   A. ac
   B. pc
   C. hs
   D. au

3. The directions for use of a medication are "Tylenol 80 mg pr q6h prn." What dosage form should be dispensed?
   A. Chew tab
   B. Syrup
   C. Suppository
   D. Enema

4. The directions for use are "Nitrostat 1/200 gr sl prn." How should this be administered?
   A. In the left ear
   B. Very slowly
   C. Under the tongue
   D. Under the skin

5. When a drug is filtered by the liver, this is referred to as
   A. Absorption
   B. Distribution
   C. Metabolism
   D. Excretion

6. Which of the following dosage forms should be stored in the refrigerator?
   A. Suppositories
   B. Patches
   C. Enemas
   D. Tablets

7. Which route of administration has the quickest onset of action?
   A. IM
   B. PR
   C. IV
   D. PO

8. The directions for use are "I gtt od qd." The medication may be
   A. Ear drops
   B. Eye drops
   C. Suppositories
   D. Vaginal tablets

9. The abbreviation *NGT* refers to
   A. Nitroglycerin
   B. Nothing by gastrostomy tube
   C. Nasal gastric
   D. Nasal gastric tube

10. The pharmaceutical abbreviation *CD* refers to
    A. Controlled drug
    B. Compact disk
    C. Controlled diffusion
    D. Continuous drip

11. A suspension should always have which auxiliary label?
    A. Keep refrigerated
    B. Shake well
    C. For external use only
    D. May cause drowsiness

Copyright © 2007 Elsevier, Inc. All rights reserved.

## MATCHING

### Matching I

Match the following abbreviations with their meanings.

| | | |
|---|---|---|
| ____ 1. AD | A. | Intravenous |
| ____ 2. OU | B. | Left eye |
| ____ 3. SQ | C. | Intradermal |
| ____ 4. IV | D. | By mouth |
| ____ 5. AS | E. | Right ear |
| ____ 6. IVPB | F. | Subcutaneous |
| ____ 7. OS | G. | Intramuscular |
| ____ 8. IM | H. | Both eyes |
| ____ 9. PO | I. | Left ear |
| ____ 10. ID | J. | Intravenous piggyback |

### Matching II

| | | |
|---|---|---|
| 1. ____ Solid | A. | Elixir |
| 2. ____ Liquid | B. | Transdermal medication |
| 3. ____ Semisolid | C. | Rectal/vaginal |
| 4. ____ Ocular | D. | Evacuation of intestines |
| 5. ____ Implant | E. | Absorb skin secretions |
| 6. ____ Patches | F. | Eye lenses |
| 7. ____ Inhalant | G. | Tablet |
| 8. ____ Enema | H. | Lotion |
| 9. ____ Paste | I. | Nebulizer |
| 10. ____ Suppositories | J. | Special capsule |

## FILL IN THE BLANK

1. What type of tablet is best for children? _____

2. Three types of capsules are _____, _____, and _____.

3. What are two uses for patches? _____ and _____

4. Syrups are _____ based, and elixirs are _____ based.

5. Suppositories may be administered _____ or _____.

6. The most commonly used SL tablet is _____.

7. Topical agents work at the _____ _____ _____.

8. The last phase of a drug's life in the body is _____.

9. All types of dosage forms manufactured must be approved by the _____.

10. Name four types of semisolids: _____, _____, _____, and _____

## SHORT ANSWER

1. Describe the "first-pass" effect of drugs in the liver.

_____

_____

_____

2. How are medications packaged?

_____

_____

_____

Copyright © 2007 Elsevier, Inc. All rights reserved.

**Active Ingredients**

1. Visit a local pharmacy. Locate the cough and cold section. Select one brand of medication with the following dosage forms: tablet, capsule, and liquid. What are the active ingredients in all three dosage forms?

2. List as many dosage forms as you can. Write two advantages and two disadvantages of each.

*Example:* Tablet—advantage, easy to carry; disadvantage, tastes bad

**CRITICAL THINKING**

1. Interpreting prescriptions can be challenging because of the various handwriting styles of physicians. Think of three rules that can make this task easier.

2. Five-year-old Tommy refuses to take his medication for iron deficiency anemia. The pharmacist has tried to mask the taste by using various compounds, but none seems to work. He finally asks for your help. What would you use that would make Tommy want to take his medicine?

3. Compounding medications unavailable commercially is much like creating a good recipe in the kitchen. Compare and contrast the two tasks. How are they similar, and how do they differ?

   Copyright © 2007 Elsevier, Inc. All rights reserved.

# 6 Referencing

## TERMS AND DEFINITIONS

Select the correct term from the following list and write the corresponding letter in the blank next to the statement.

A. Chemical structure

B. Brand/trade

C. Drug classification

D. Formulary

E. Generic name

F. Monograph

G. Pharmacology

_____ 1. The study of drugs and their effects on the body

_____ 2. A list of drugs approved for use from which choices are made

_____ 3. The shape of molecules and their location with regard to one another

_____ 4. Based on the action of a drug and its use

_____ 5. The description of a drug, including side effects, dosage forms, indications, and other pertinent information

_____ 6. Trademark of a drug or device created by the original manufacturer

_____ 7. Name assigned to a medication by the FDA

## TRUE OR FALSE

Write T or F next to each statement.

_____ 1. Pharmacy reference books are used by pharmacy personnel only.

_____ 2. Pharmacists rely on good reference books to help give correct information to other health care workers.

_____ 3. Manufacturers give a drug a name based on its chemical attributes.

_____ 4. All brand, or trade, drug names should be capitalized.

_____ 5. Contraindications list the main conditions for which the drug is used.

_____ 6. All technicians should carry a *Facts and Comparisons* in their pocket.

## MULTIPLE CHOICE

Complete each question by circling the best answer.

1. The reference most often used by pharmacists is
   A. *Facts and Comparisons*
   B. *Physicians' Desk Reference*
   C. *The Red Book*
   D. *United States Pharmacopoeia*

2. The section of *Facts and Comparisons* that shows more than 250 of the most used drugs in color is the
   A. Index
   B. Drug monograph
   C. Drug identification
   D. Appendix

3. The reference book known as the *PDR* is the
   A. *Pharmacists' Drug Reference*
   B. *Physicians' Desk Reference*

   C. *Pharmacist Desk Reference*
   D. *Pharmacy Dosage Regulations*

4. The PDR contains what information?
   A. Manufacturers' addresses and phone numbers
   B. All FDA-approved drugs
   C. Products listed by classification or method of action
   D. All of the above

5. The diagnostic product information section of the PDR contains
   A. A key to controlled substances
   B. A key to FDA pregnancy ratings
   C. An FDA telephone directory
   D. Information on drug products used as diagnostic agents

Copyright © 2007 Elsevier, Inc. All rights reserved.

6. If the technician must know the upper limit price and rules on what units each type of drug must be billed on for state AIDS drug assistance programs, the technician would use
   A. *Facts and Comparisons*
   B. *Physicians' Desk Reference*
   C. *The Red Book*
   D. *Orange Book Code*

7. A patient has taken a drug but does not know what it is; the technician can use which reference book to find out what the drug is?
   A. *American Hospital Formulary Service Drug Information*
   B. *United States Pharmacopoeia Drug Information*
   C. *Ident-A-Drug*
   D. *The Injectable Drug Handbook*

8. The book used to reference the compatibility of various agents being given parenterally is
   A. *American Hospital Formulary Service Drug Information*
   B. *United States Pharmacopoeia Drug Information*
   C. *Ident-A-Drug*
   D. *The Injectable Drug Handbook*

9. *Facts and Comparisons* is updated
   A. Monthly
   B. Yearly
   C. A and B
   D. None of the above

10. Pharmacy journals contain information about
    A. New drugs
    B. The future of pharmacy
    C. Legislative changes
    D. All of the above

11. Currently, only one association is run by technicians and allows only technicians as members. It is the
    A. NPTA
    B. AAPT
    C. ASHP
    D. APhA

12. The reference book needed to find a sugar-free and alcohol-free cough syrup is the
    A. *Physicians' Desk Reference*
    B. *Red Book*
    C. *Facts and Comparisons*
    D. *Ident-A-Drug*

## MATCHING

**Matching I**

____ 1. FDA

____ 2. Monographs

____ 3. Contraindications

____ 4. Indications

____ 5. Classification

A. Package inserts

B. Identifies the types of people who should not be given the drug

C. Approves all new drugs

D. Puts drugs into the proper category based on chemical actions

E. Lists main conditions for which a chemical is used

**Matching II**

____ 1. UPC

____ 2. AWP

____ 3. NDC

____ 4. USP

____ 5. F&C

A. Average wholesale price

B. *Facts and Comparisons*

C. *U.S. Pharmacopeia*

D. Universal Product Code

E. National Drug Code

## FILL IN THE BLANK

1. _____ is the reference text most often used in pharmacies.

2. The reference text most often used in a physician's office is the _____.

3. The _____ book is a good source of information on drug costs.

4. The _____ book is a comprehensive listing of approved drug products with therapeutic equivalent evaluations.

5. A comprehensive listing of approved formulary drugs, their uses, and adverse reactions that is used primarily in the hospital is the _____.

Copyright © 2007 Elsevier, Inc. All rights reserved.

## RESEARCH ACTIVITY

1. Access the websites listed in Table 6-6 of the textbook. Describe the type of information provided on each website.

## CRITICAL THINKING

1. Of all the reference books discussed in the chapter, which one seems to be the easiest to use and understand?

2. Think of some of the magazines you have read or glanced through on a newsstand lately. How many of them included some sort of medical, drug, or health-related article or information? Did the articles spark your interest? If so, why? Were any of them written by professionals in the field?

3. List as many sources as possible that could be used as resources for drug information and that can be accessed without having to buy a book on the subject.

Copyright © 2007 Elsevier, Inc. All rights reserved.

# 7 Competency, Communication, and Ethics

## TERMS AND DEFINITIONS

Select the correct term from the following list and write the corresponding letter in the blank next to the statement.

A. Communication

B. Confidentiality

C. Ethics

D. Professionalism

_____ 1. Keeping privileged information about a customer from being disclosed without the person's consent

_____ 2. The ability to express oneself in such a way that one is readily and clearly understood

_____ 3. The values and morals used within a profession

_____ 4. Conforming to right principles of conduct (work ethics) as accepted by others in the profession

## TRUE OR FALSE

Write T or F next to each statement.

_____ 1. As the population grows older, the use of prescription medications continues to grow.

_____ 2. Each state has its own board of pharmacy, which establishes regulations for pharmacy technicians.

_____ 3. Meeting state-specific guidelines is the least basic requirement for a pharmacy technician.

_____ 4. Knowledge of pharmacy law is not essential to work in a pharmacy environment.

_____ 5. Pharmacists can and will catch every mistake a pharmacy technician makes.

_____ 6. Pharmacies regularly take samples of compounded IVs and send them to the laboratory to be tested for microbial growth.

_____ 7. Drugs that look alike or have names that sound alike have been the cause of many pharmacy errors.

_____ 8. Pharmacy technicians are taking over the traditional role of the pharmacist.

_____ 9. The term *communication skills* refers to verbal skills only.

_____ 10. Allowing patients to express their frustrations, being a good listener, and doing one's best to help people are what being a professional is all about.

## MULTIPLE CHOICE

Complete the question by circling the best answer.

1. Which of the following is the top cause of injury and death in the United States?
   A. Medication errors
   B. Breast cancer
   C. Motor vehicle accidents
   D. AIDS

2. When consumers or people in the medical community want to report a medication error, they can contact
   A. *Ident-A-Drug*
   B. *Med Watch*
   C. *Facts and Comparisons*
   D. *Consumer Reports*

3. One way to reduce the number of errors is to
   A. Shelve drugs alphabetically by generic name
   B. Let the pharmacist fill all orders
   C. Read medication labels three times
   D. Ask the patient to check the drug

4. What factors must be considered before a person can be considered a competent pharmacy technician?
   A. Job duties
   B. Communication skills
   C. Ethics
   D. All of the above

**27**

Copyright © 2007 Elsevier, Inc. All rights reserved.

5. Which of the following is considered a way of communicating?
   A. Speaking
   B. Listening
   C. Body language
   D. All of the above

6. Which of the following is *not* considered part of a technician's professional appearance?
   A. Wedding ring
   B. Earring
   C. Nose ring
   D. Engagement ring

7. The daily duties of a pharmacy technician include
   A. Answering phones
   B. Taking messages
   C. Talking to nurses
   D. All of the above

8. Working ethically is
   A. Doing what is right for your beliefs
   B. Doing what is right for the patient
   C. Giving the patient everything the person wants
   D. Showing up for work on time every day

9. Pharmacy technicians have access to confidential information, such as
   A. Medical conditions
   B. Vehicle identification number
   C. Driver's license number
   D. All of the above

10. Terminally ill patients go through five stages
    A. Starting with anger, ending with depression
    B. Starting with denial, ending with acceptance
    C. Starting with anger, ending with acceptance
    D. Starting with denial, ending with depression

## EXPLAIN

1. Why is registration such an important tool for pharmacy management?

_____

_____

_____

2. To what does the policy and procedure (P&P) of each pharmacy pertain?

_____

_____

_____

3. Give three common reasons medication errors occur.

   A. _____

   B. _____

   C. _____

4. What three traits must a person have to be considered a professional?

   A. _____

   B. _____

   C. _____

5. Define *confidentiality*. _____

_____

## ABBREVIATIONS

Give the abbreviation for the following agencies.

_____ 1. Federal Drug Administration

_____ 2. Joint Commission on Accreditation of Hospital Organizations

_____ 3. American Society of Health-System Pharmacists

_____ 4. Center for Drug Evaluation and Research

**28**

Chapter **7** **Competency, Communication, and Ethics**

Copyright © 2007 Elsevier, Inc. All rights reserved.

## FILL IN THE BLANK

1. _____ and _____ help pharmacy management more easily choose the most competent technician to fill the position.

2. A _____ is a job, occupation, or line of work that becomes a career.

3. Good communication skills include _____, _____, _____, _____, _____, and _____.

4. Pharmacy protocol usually outlines what is _____ and _____ with regard to appearance.

5. The pharmacy technician can influence the development of a _____ atmosphere in the pharmacy setting.

## RESEARCH ACTIVITY

Access the Internet. Using the search engine *www.google.com*, locate the websites for the agencies included in the Abbreviations section and list them here.

1. _____

2. _____

3. _____

4. _____

## CRITICAL THINKING

1. What do you know about the pharmacy technician's scope of practice (i.e., what the technician is/is not allowed to do) in your state?

2. What does your state Practice Act require of pharmacy technicians?

3. Why is it so important for you to become a certified pharmacy technician? Give at least five reasons.

4. Mastering competencies is very important for pharmacy technicians. What five competencies would you like to master as a technician? Why?

5. Everyone is guided and shaped by a code of ethics and morality. Think of the guidelines (do's/don'ts) you grew up with and develop your own code of ethics. What do you live by? How important is it to develop a good work ethic? What three important character traits do employers seek in an employee?

Copyright © 2007 Elsevier, Inc. All rights reserved.

# 8 Prescription Processing

**TERMS AND DEFINITIONS**

## TERMS AND DEFINITIONS

Select the correct term from the following list and write the corresponding letter in the blank next to the statement.

A. Auxiliary label

B. Inpatient pharmacy

C. Hard copy

D. Adjudication

E. OTC

F. Outpatient pharmacy

G. RTS

H. RX

I. Script

J. Sig

_____ 1. Return to stock

_____ 2. A prescription

_____ 3. A hospital or institutional pharmacy

_____ 4. Over-the-counter

_____ 5. The electronic determination whether a person's insurance coverage is confirmed

_____ 6. The original prescription

_____ 7. Latin for "recipe"; commonly used to mean "prescription"

_____ 8. A community pharmacy

_____ 9. An adhesive label that is attached to a container with specific instructions or information pertaining to the medication inside

_____ 10. Medication directions written in pharmacy terms on a prescription

## TRUE OR FALSE

Write T or F next to each statement.

_____ 1. One of the most important duties performed by a technician is filling prescriptions.

_____ 2. If technicians cannot interpret the information on a prescription, they should quickly make an educated guess.

_____ 3. Five basic steps are involved in filling a prescription, and all five relate directly to the technician.

_____ 4. The person at the take-in counter is the first one to handle the script.

_____ 5. If a prescription is filled by a technician incorrectly, the outcome affects only the technician who filled the order.

_____ 6. Most court cases favor the pharmacist and award the pharmacy cash settlements.

_____ 7. All vials leaving the pharmacy must, by law, have childproof lids.

_____ 8. The technician should check the medication against the script and the label when selecting medication from the shelf.

_____ 9. The prescription label must show the name, address, and phone number of the pharmacy.

_____ 10. The last step in filling prescriptions is to pass the prescription to the pharmacist for final inspection and signature.

## MULTIPLE CHOICE

Complete the question by circling the best answer.

1. When taking in a prescription, neither the technician nor the pharmacist can decipher the doctor's writing; therefore
   A. The technician should guess what to fill
   B. The technician should ask the patient
   C. The pharmacist should call the physician
   D. The technician should tell the patient to go back to the doctor and get a prescription that can be read

Copyright © 2007 Elsevier, Inc. All rights reserved.

2. Which of the following is not the duty of a technician in taking in a prescription?
   A. Translating the prescription
   B. Entering information into the database
   C. Filling the prescription
   D. Providing patient consultation

3. When a new prescription is called in to the pharmacy, who can take the prescription over the phone?
   A. Pharmacy clerk
   B. Pharmacy technician
   C. Pharmacist
   D. Pharmacy custodian

4. If a prescription is for a narcotic, the technician must make sure the prescription has the physician's
   A. FDA number
   B. DEA number
   C. HMO number
   D. NABP number

5. Most dosing in an inpatient pharmacy is set for a _____ period.
   A. 12 hour
   B. 24 hour
   C. 36 hour
   D. 48 hour

6. Which of the following is *not* an exception to the safety lid law?
   A. Nitroglycerin
   B. Patient's request
   C. Isosorbide SL
   D. Technician's opinion that the patient looks too weak to open a safety lid

7. Which of the following is *not* preprinted on a label as required by law?
   A. Name, address, and phone number of prescriber
   B. Prescription number
   C. Drug, strength, and dosage form
   D. Refill information

8. Which of the following is *not* a common auxiliary label for narcotics?
   A. May cause drowsiness/dizziness
   B. May cause sensitivity to light
   C. Do not drink alcohol
   D. Alcohol may increase the effects of the drug

9. Which of the following is *not* an advantage of computer-dispensing systems?
   A. They have a high cost
   B. They increase productivity
   C. They cut down on errors
   D. They allow for better inventory control

10. The law states that all prescriptions must be kept on file for at least
    A. 6 months
    B. 1 year
    C. 3 years
    D. 5 years

11. Prescriptions that have a red "C" stamped on the right side indicate that the prescription is for
    A. A controlled substance
    B. A cough medication
    C. A drug containing codeine
    D. A cardiac medication

12. Pharmacy technicians must be capable of
    A. Interpreting and transcribing prescriptions
    B. Filling prescriptions quickly and accurately
    C. Following proper billing practices
    D. All of the above

13. According to federal law, when should a patient receive counseling?
    A. At the last refill of the patient's medication
    B. Only when the patient asks for it
    C. When a new prescription is filled
    D. At all times

14. Most boards of pharmacy prefer to allow transfer of prescriptions only _____ time(s).
    A. One
    B. Two
    C. Three
    D. 0

## EXPLAIN

1. When you check the label against the script, for what are you checking?

_____

_____

2. Why do older patients not want safety lids on their medications?

_____

_____

3. Why should technicians initial any prescriptions they fill?

_____

_____

   Copyright © 2007 Elsevier, Inc. All rights reserved.

## SHORT ANSWER

1. List the five rights of the patient

   A. _____

   B. _____

   C. _____

   D. _____

   E. _____

2. List the five steps of processing a prescription.

   A. _____

   B. _____

   C. _____

   D. _____

   E. _____

3. What should be checked before a prescription is released to a relative?

   A. _____

   B. _____

4. What are the "meat and potatoes" of pharmacy?

   _____

   _____

## RESEARCH ACTIVITY

Access the websites *www.pyxis.com* and *www.mckesson.co*m.

1. Look up news and events. What is the latest in automated technology/products in development for pharmacies?

2. How many different products for automation are there?

## CRITICAL THINKING

1. Give five differences in handling prescriptions/medication orders between the outpatient and the inpatient setting.

2. You have received a medication order for a chemotherapy drug in the pharmacy. You are the technician preparing chemotherapy when the order comes in by fax. You are not sure what the drug is on the order, so you consult the pharmacist. After some discussion, the two of you decide what the drug is, and the order is prepared. Who else would be able to verify that this is the correct medication before it is administered to the patient?

Copyright © 2007 Elsevier, Inc. All rights reserved.

3. After filling about 25 prescriptions on a very busy morning in the pharmacy, you realize that you might have made a mistake on the last one. It is time to go to lunch, so you decide to let it go, believing that the pharmacist will catch it. Unfortunately, the pharmacist checks the prescription hurriedly, trusting that you did your job correctly, and the prescription goes home with the patient.
   A. What should you have done to prevent this medication error?
   B. Whose fault is it that the prescription was dispensed as is?
   C. What can you do to remedy the situation before the patient is harmed by your mistake?

Copyright © 2007 Elsevier, Inc. All rights reserved.

# 9 Over-the-Counter Medications and Skin Care Products

**TERMS AND DEFINITIONS**

Select the correct term from the following list and write the corresponding letter in the blank next to the statement.

A. Analgesic

B. Antiinflammatory

C. Antipruritic

D. Antiseptic

E. Antitussive

F. ASA

G. Bulk forming

H. Desquamating

I. Expectorant

J. Keratolytic

K. OTC

L. Protectant

M. Prophylaxis

N. Pruritus

O. ROA

P. RX

Q. Sunscreen

_____ 1. A substance that stops or slows the growth of microorganisms on surfaces such as skin

_____ 2. An over-the-counter medication; does not require a prescription

_____ 3. Routes of administration

_____ 4. A medication that causes loss of sensation/pain due to an interruption in the nervous system pathway between the organ and the brain

_____ 5. Aspirin

_____ 6. Itching

_____ 7. A drug that induces the patient to cough up mucus from the lungs

_____ 8. A substance that protects the skin from ultraviolet (UV) light, which causes sunburns; skin protection factor (SPF) rates effectiveness

_____ 9. The normal process of shedding of the top layer of skin; also known as *exfoliation*

_____ 10. A drug that reduces swelling, redness, and pain and promotes healing

_____ 11. A substance that acts as a barrier between the skin and an irritant

_____ 12. A drug that relieves itching; usually an antihistamine or an antiinflammatory drug

_____ 13. A drug that causes shedding of the outer layer of the skin

_____ 14. A legend drug; a drug that requires a prescription

_____ 15. Fiber used as a stimulant to the intestines or to cause a feeling of fullness to reduce appetite

_____ 16. Treatment given before a possible event to prevent the event from happening

_____ 17. A drug that can reduce the coughing reflex of the CNS

Copyright © 2007 Elsevier, Inc. All rights reserved.

## TRUE OR FALSE

Write T or F next to each statement.

_____ 1. The ability to buy drugs over the counter can be a substantial savings for customers.

_____ 2. Most OTC drugs do recommend dosages for children younger than 2 years.

_____ 3. Adverse reaction reports are required for both prescription and OTC drugs.

_____ 4. Very few agents are 100% pure.

_____ 5. The *potency* of a medication refers to the strength of the drug.

_____ 6. *Bioavailability* is the amount of drug available from the manufacturer.

_____ 7. *Efficacy* is the ability of the drug to produce the desired effect in the body.

_____ 8. The standards of safety and effectiveness are lower for OTC drugs than for legend drugs.

_____ 9. Sunburn and acne are very serious skin conditions and should not be treated at home.

_____ 10. Strep throat can be treated with OTC medications

## MULTIPLE CHOICE

Complete each question by circling the best answer.

1. The number of OTC drugs available to consumers has increased since the
   A. 1960s
   B. 1970s
   C. 1980s
   D. 1990s

2. Drug companies know that consumers want more OTC drugs available to them so that they can
   A. Save money
   B. Be involved in their own treatment
   C. Both A and B
   D. None of the above

3. Which of the following is *not* a category applied by the FDA to rate OTC drugs before they are allowed to enter the market?
   A. Safe and effective for the claimed therapeutic indication
   B. Not recognized as safe and effective
   C. Additional data need to be obtained to determine safety and efficacy
   D. Toxic; no additional data needed

4. The FDA regulates aspects affecting the safety of OTC medications; the aspects regulated are
   A. Purity and potency
   B. Bioavailability and efficacy
   C. Safety and toxicity
   D. All of the above

5. New OTC drugs must go through certain phases before approval. The phase during which a final review is done on the ingredients of the drug and the public is allowed to give feedback is known as
   A. Phase 1
   B. Phase 2
   C. Phase 3
   D. Phase 4

6. A *monograph* is
   A. Information about a drug
   B. Descriptive information about clinical trials
   C. A picture of the chemical compound of the drug
   D. A and B

7. Which condition cannot be treated with OTC drugs?
   A. High blood pressure
   B. Fever
   C. Cough
   D. Diarrhea

8. Children and teenagers should not take aspirin for chickenpox or flu, because it has been associated with
   A. Toxic shock syndrome
   B. Reye's syndrome
   C. Sudden infant death syndrome
   D. Acquired immunodeficiency syndrome

9. *NSAID* stands for
   A. Nonsafety caps for AIDS patients
   B. Not safe as an IUD service
   C. Nonsteroidal antiinflammatory drug
   D. Nonsteroidal antiinflammatory disease

10. A common side effect of first-generation antihistamines is
    A. Drowsiness
    B. Diarrhea
    C. Agitation
    D. Constipation

Copyright © 2007 Elsevier, Inc. All rights reserved.

11. What is the largest organ of the body?
   A. Heart
   B. Lungs
   C. Kidneys
   D. Skin

12. Which of the following noninfectious skin conditions is *not* an allergic reaction?
   A. Atopic dermatitis
   B. Psoriasis
   C. Eczema
   D. Urticaria

## SHORT ANSWER

1. Give three examples of antiinflammatory products.

   A. _____

   B. _____

   C. _____

2. Which decongestant does not cause drowsiness? _____

3. What is the most commonly prescribed agent used in hospitals to help patients sleep?
   _____

4. Give two classes of drugs used to reduce or relieve acid secretions.

   A. _____

   B. _____

5. Into which layer of skin does a diabetic person inject insulin? _____

6. How do sunscreens and sun blocks work?

   A. Sunscreens _____
   _____

   B. Sun blocks _____
   _____

7. What is the most common OTC product recommended to help dry out pimples?
   _____

8. The only treatment for acne is to _____
   _____

9. A. What is psoriasis? B. How is it treated?

   A. _____
   _____

   B. _____
   _____

## MATCHING

Match the term in the left column with the alternative name in the right column.

| | | |
|---|---|---|
| _____ 1. Urticaria | A. Herpes simplex virus |
| _____ 2. Genital warts | B. Small topical ulcers |
| _____ 3. Tinea pedis | C. Hives |
| _____ 4. Canker sores | D. Human papillomavirus |
| _____ 5. Cold sores | E. Athlete's foot |

Copyright © 2007 Elsevier, Inc. All rights reserved.

**RESEARCH ACTIVITY**

1. Access the website *www.fda.gov*. In the Quick Info Links section, locate Drugs@FDA; type in OTC. Investigate what legend drugs have been converted to OTC status.

2. Access the website *www.accutanehelp.com*.
   A. What are some of the serious side effects of the acne product Accutane?
   B. What precautions should be taken by patients using this skin care product?

**CRITICAL THINKING**

1. In a chain store or mass merchandiser outlet, where is the pharmacy located? Why?

2. You have a sore throat, and none of the OTC lozenges are helping. You have been told to gargle with saltwater. How will this help your sore throat?

3. Sometimes a person buys an OTC medication because someone they know tried it and it worked for that person. Why should you not base your decision to buy OTC medications on that reasoning?

4. The FDA recently allowed Prilosec to become an OTC product. What other drugs do you think should become OTC medications, providing they are safe and effective for patients?

5. Tanning beds, airbrushed tans, and tans in a bottle are very popular products. What are the dangers of overusing some of these products on your skin? What advice would you give people you know who are overusing these products?

Copyright © 2007 Elsevier, Inc. All rights reserved.

# 10 Complementary Alternative Medicine

## TERMS AND DEFINITIONS

Select the correct term from the following list and write the corresponding letter in the blank next to the statement.

A. Antiemetic

B. Antihypertensive

C. Ayurveda

D. Chiropractic

E. Diagnosis

F. Fat-soluble

G. Herbs

H. Homeopathy

I. Legend drug

J. OTC

K. Placebo

L. Synthetic

M. Tinctures

_____ 1. An inert compound thought to be an active agent

_____ 2. A holistic medical system that originated in India

_____ 3. A system of therapy based on the belief that medicinal substances that cause a specific symptom can be used to treat an illness that yields the same symptoms

_____ 4. A doctor's assessment of the cause of a condition

_____ 5. Drugs that are absorbed into the body's fat layer

_____ 6. Plant extract mixed with alcohol

_____ 7. Manual manipulation of the joints and muscles

_____ 8. Agents that stop nausea and vomiting

_____ 9. Over-the-counter medications

_____ 10. Medication that requires a prescription

_____ 11. Medication made in a laboratory

_____ 12. Agents that reduce blood pressure

_____ 13. Any herbaceous plant consisting of fleshy stems

## TRUE OR FALSE

Write T or F next to each statement.

_____ 1. Traditional medicine has been in existence for thousands of years, whereas alternative approaches have been practiced for only a few hundred years.

_____ 2. Western medicine relies on scientific methods to prove the effectiveness of treatments.

_____ 3. Developing countries use herbs as their main form of treatment.

_____ 4. Herbs are considered a form of traditional medication.

_____ 5. Self-hypnosis was found clinically to reduce the pain of surgery in patients.

_____ 6. A placebo contains no active ingredients.

_____ 7. Biofeedback should be practiced only with a biofeedback instructor present.

_____ 8. Chiropractic therapy usually requires many treatment sessions.

_____ 9. Crystal healing is a well-documented, scientific study of overcoming illnesses.

_____ 10. Herbs are natural and therefore not harmful.

_____ 11. Herbs that are brewed for teas usually are more potent than those prepared in capsule form.

_____ 12. Many physicians and scientists consider spiritual healing a testimonial to the power of the placebo effect.

Copyright © 2007 Elsevier, Inc. All rights reserved.

## MULTIPLE CHOICE

Complete the question by circling the best answer.

1. Traditional medicine includes all of the following except
   A. Doctor visits
   B. Prescription drugs
   C. Laboratory tests
   D. Visits to a chiropractor

2. Complementary alternative medicine includes all of the following except
   A. Herbs
   B. X-rays
   C. Acupuncture
   D. Yoga

3. Controversial therapies include
   A. Crystal healing
   B. Spiritual healing
   C. Magnetic healing
   D. All of the above

4. Eastern medicine includes treatments originating from all of the following except
   A. Eastern Asia
   B. India
   C. Eastern United States
   D. Far East countries

5. The beginning of the golden age of microbiology is considered to be the
   A. 1600s
   B. 1700s
   C. 1800s
   D. 1900s

6. A reason people may turn to alternative medicines is
   A. Risk of drug side effects
   B. Rising cost of drugs
   C. Diseases for which no medications are available
   D. All of the above

7. Which of the following is *not* considered a nondrug treatment?
   A. Massage
   B. Herbs
   C. Meditation
   D. Biofeedback

8. Herbs used in Chinese medicine can
   A. Cure the body of illness
   B. Prevent future problems
   C. A and B
   D. None of the above

9. Biofeedback has been proved to be effective for all of the following *except*
   A. Love life
   B. Heart rate
   C. Hypertension
   D. Gastrointestinal activity

10. Chiropractic treatment can include all of the following *except*
    A. Adjustments of the joints
    B. Chemotherapy
    C. Massage
    D. Heat therapy

11. To treat a minor burn, a patient could use
    A. Aloe vera
    B. Chamomile
    C. Garlic
    D. Gingko biloba

12. The belief that if a small amount of the substance that caused a person's disease or condition is consumed, it will enable the body to fight off the disease is known as
    A. The placebo effect
    B. Ayurveda
    C. Homeopathy
    D. Spiritual healing

## FILL IN THE BLANK

1. From which plant is the heart drug digoxin made? _____

2. What form of alternative medicine uses needles inserted at specific points throughout the body?
   _____

3. The heart of Chinese medicine is the _____ and _____, which represent both _____ and _____ entities.

4. Art therapy is used extensively in _____ with _____.

5. Ayurveda is based on the person knowing his or her _____ _____.

6. Chiropractic therapy is an _____ approach to treating pain from _____ of bones.

7. The FDA does not regulate herbs because they are considered to be _____
   _____.

Copyright © 2007 Elsevier, Inc. All rights reserved.

## MATCHING

Match the following herbs with their treatment targets.

| | | | |
|---|---|---|---|
| ____ 1. Black cohosh | A. Sleep |
| ____ 2. Chamomile | B. Overall wellness |
| ____ 3. Ginger | C. Colds and infections |
| ____ 4. Milk thistle | D. Depression and fatigue |
| ____ 5. Echinacea | E. Motion sickness, flatulence, gastrointestinal disturbances |
| ____ 6. Garlic | F. Poor circulation |
| ____ 7. Ginkgo biloba | G. Antiemetic, vertigo |
| ____ 8. Ginseng | H. Liver conditions |
| ____ 9. St. John's Wort | I. Hormone replacement |
| ____ 10. Valerian | J. Hypertension, high cholesterol |

## EXPLAIN

1. Why is it important to know the family name of an herb? _____

_____

2. What is the premise of homeopathy? _____

_____

## SHORT ANSWER

1. The holistic approach to diagnosis and treatments includes _____, _____, and even _____.

2. What are the three main goals of NCCAM?

   A. _____

   B. _____

   C. _____

3. Complementary medicine is the use of _____therapies and _____ medicine together.

4. Who oversees the manufacture of homeopathic drugs? _____.

5. Homeopathic drugs are in the same category as _____ drugs.

## RESEARCH ACTIVITY

1. Access the website *www.rxlist.com*. Locate the list, Top 30 Western Herbs. Print the list and compare the various herbs and treatments with those discussed in the chapter.

2. Access the website *www.altmedicine.com*. What is the purpose of this website?

Copyright © 2007 Elsevier, Inc. All rights reserved.

Chapter **10** **Complementary Alternative Medicine**

3. Access the website *http://nccam.nih.gov/health*. Read the information given under Understanding Complementary and Alternative Medicine (CAM).

## CRITICAL THINKING

1. Alternative medicine has been on the rise the past few years. Many people are not aware that the FDA does not regulate many of the "natural" products being marketed. As a consumer, how can you be sure that these "natural" products really contain the ingredients reported on the labels?

2. Besides the various therapies and herbal products discussed in the chapter, what other forms of alternative medicine are available?

3. Spiritual healing brings another dimension to alternative medicine. Why is it so different from the other forms discussed in the chapter?

4. You are trying to convince your classmates that trying alternative medicine is better than seeing a physician every time you feel ill. How would you make your case for this form of therapy?

Copyright © 2007 Elsevier, Inc. All rights reserved.

# 11 Hospital Pharmacy

## TERMS AND DEFINITIONS

Select the correct term from the following list and write the corresponding letter in the blank next to the statement.

A. Aseptic technique

B. Floor stock

C. Inpatient

D. MAR

E. NKDA

F. On-call

G. Pre-op

H. PRN

I. Protocol

J. Stat order

_____ 1. No known drug allergy

_____ 2. A set of standards and guidelines by which the facility works

_____ 3. A drug ordered to be given before surgery

_____ 4. As needed

_____ 5. Medication administration record

_____ 6. When a medication is written for preanesthesia and will be used when needed

_____ 7. A hospitalized patient

_____ 8. A method of preventing contamination by organisms

_____ 9. Must be filled as soon as possible, usually within 5 to 15 minutes

_____ 10. Supplies kept on hand in different units of the hospital

## TRUE OR FALSE

Write T or F next to each statement.

_____ 1. A hospital pharmacy is one of the most challenging areas in which a pharmacy technician can work.

_____ 2. Hospital pharmacies have more job openings than community pharmacies.

_____ 3. Large hospitals may have a central pharmacy and smaller satellite pharmacies throughout the hospital.

_____ 4. Satellite pharmacies stock specific medications for the ward they service to speed up the turnaround time on medication orders.

_____ 5. All hospitals must meet only state guidelines.

_____ 6. The board of pharmacy has the authority to impose fines and to close down pharmacies.

_____ 7. Technicians must have scheduling flexibility, because they will need to work all shifts, including weekends and holidays.

_____ 8. The chemo hood normally is larger than a horizontal hood because of the additional equipment needed in the hood.

_____ 9. A hospital pharmacy must stock a wide variety of medications in many dosage forms.

_____ 10. When nurses call the pharmacy, the most common question is, "Where are the meds I ordered?"

_____ 11. Automated systems used in hospitals are replacing technicians.

_____ 12. A hospital pharmacy technician should be an energetic, multitasking-type person.

Copyright © 2007 Elsevier, Inc. All rights reserved.

## MULTIPLE CHOICE

Complete each question by circling the best answer.

1. The policies and procedures handbook contains information about
   A. Mandatory training
   B. Cafeteria menus
   C. Doctors' orders
   D. All of the above

2. *JCAHO* stands for
   A. Joint Commission about Hospital Orderlies
   B. Jewish-Catholic Association of Healthcare Organizations
   C. Joint Commission on Accreditation of Hospital Operations
   D. Joint Commission on Accreditation of Healthcare Organizations

3. One of the agencies that govern the operations of hospitals is the
   A. HFC
   B. HCFA
   C. RPH
   D. ICU

4. Which of the following is *not* a way orders arrive at the inpatient pharmacy?
   A. Fax machine
   B. Pneumatic tube
   C. Delivery by patients
   D. Delivery by staff

5. When patients with the same last name end up on the same floor, which auxiliary label should be used?
   A. Take as directed
   B. Name alert
   C. May cause drowsiness
   D. Shake well

6. IV medication order labels show the
   A. Drug name, strength, and dosage form
   B. Route of administration and scheduled dosing time
   C. Patient's name, medical record number, and room number
   D. All of the above

7. The technician responsible for filling med drawers for all current patients in the hospital is called the
   A. IV technician
   B. Satellite technician
   C. Unit-dose cart fill technician
   D. Floor stock technician

8. In a horizontal flow hood, the airflow pattern is in what direction?
   A. From the back of the hood to the front
   B. From the top of the hood to the bottom
   C. From the bottom of the hood to the top
   D. From the front of the hood to the back

9. The inventory control technician is not responsible for
   A. Computer order entry
   B. Checking off other technicians' work
   C. Billing
   D. Restocking shelves

10. Which of the following is *not* an automated hospital system?
    A. PYXIS
    B. SureMed
    C. Robot RX
    D. JCAHO

## FILL IN THE BLANK

1. _____ technique is extremely important is preparing all IV medications, _____ _____, and compounded ophthalmics.

2. When preparing chemotherapy, a technician must wear a _____ and _____ gloves.

3. The proper placement of labels is important to _____ _____ of the _____ and its contents.

4. All narcotics are counted _____ times daily on the nursing units.

5. The _____ levels are the amounts of medications that should be kept on the floor at all times.

6. Only _____ can sign in narcotics.

7. _____ is a term used to define the guidelines in a hospital setting, such as the type of medication available for dispensing.

8. Specialty technician tasks include assisting with _____ _____ and _____ therapy.

9. If the hospital uses an automated medication dispensing system, there is no need for a _____.

Copyright © 2007 Elsevier, Inc. All rights reserved.

10. The three types of STAT trays stocked by hospital pharmacies are _____, _____, and _____.

## SHORT ANSWER

1. List three duties of the inventory control technician.

   A. _____

   B. _____

   C. _____

2. What three specialty departments stock many drugs in injectable forms, as well as a variety of oral and injectable narcotics?

   A. _____

   B. _____

   C. _____

3. Stat orders can be filled in _____ minutes and if possible be _____ _____ to ensure that they get to the correct destination _____ and _____.

4. When a technician is working inside a horizontal flow hood, the orientation of the hands _____

   _____

5. For what are the following governmental agencies responsible?

   A. JCAHO _____

   B. HCFA _____

   C. BOP _____

## RESEARCH ACTIVITY

1. Access *www.ptcb.org* and look up the duties of a hospital technician.



2. Visit or call a local hospital pharmacy and interview the following hospital technicians: IV therapy, chemotherapy, UD fill, and narcotics. Ask the following questions:
   A. What are your job duties?
   B. What training did you receive?
   C. What is the most satisfying part of your job?



## CRITICAL THINKING

1. Many technicians work in inpatient hospital pharmacies because the pay scale is higher than that found in retail or community pharmacies. What are some other reasons a technician might want to work in an inpatient hospital pharmacy?

Copyright © 2007 Elsevier, Inc. All rights reserved.

2. The job descriptions of inpatient pharmacy technicians are changing because of the various automated systems coming into use to fill medication carts. Outline a job description for an automated dispensing technician.

3. The relationship between the nursing and pharmacy staffs can be tumultuous at times. How can you, as a technician, foster a better relationship between these two groups of professionals?

Copyright © 2007 Elsevier, Inc. All rights reserved.

# 12 Repackaging and Compounding

## TERMS AND DEFINITIONS

Select the correct term from the following list and write the corresponding letter in the blank next to the statement.

A. Blister packs

B. Bulk compounding

C. Calibration

D. Compounding

E. Cream

F. Elixir

G. FDA

H. Hydrophilic

I. Hydrophobic

J. Mortar and pestle

K. Ointment

L. Reconstitution

M. Repackaging

N. Solute

O. Solution

P. Solvent

Q. Suspension

R. Syrup

S. Tincture

T. Unit-dose

U. Monthly supply

_____ 1. To mix a liquid and a powder to form a suspension or solution

_____ 2. Water loving; any substance that easily dissolves in water

_____ 3. A solution in which solid particles do not dissolve into the base, requiring the solution to be shaken before use

_____ 4. The act of mixing, reconstituting, and packaging a drug

_____ 5. A larger quantity of medication that can fill a large order at one time or several smaller orders in the future

_____ 6. Typically a 30-day supply

_____ 7. A bowl and rounded knob used to grind substances into fine powder

_____ 8. The act of reducing the amount of medication taken from a bulk bottle; unit dosing

_____ 9. A single dose of a drug

_____ 10. A base solution that is a mixture of alcohol and water

_____ 11. The ingredient that is dissolved into a solution

_____ 12. A sugar-based liquid

_____ 13. Food and Drug Administration

_____ 14. Containers, usually made of plastic, that hold a single-dose tablet or capsule

_____ 15. A base solution of alcohol

_____ 16. The markings on a measuring device

_____ 17. A water base in which the ingredients dissolve completely

_____ 18. A hydrophilic base

_____ 19. Water hating; any substance that does not dissolve in water

_____ 20. The greater part of a solution

_____ 21. A hydrophobic product, such as Vaseline

Copyright © 2007 Elsevier, Inc. All rights reserved.

## TRUE OR FALSE

Write T or F next to each statement.

_____ 1. Repackaging of medication is a common process in a hospital pharmacy.

_____ 2. No expiration date is necessary for repackaged products.

_____ 3. The process of repackaging should be done in a horizontal flow hood.

_____ 4. If the expiration date includes the month and year, the drug expires on the first day of the month.

_____ 5. Part of the preparation for repackaging is accurate calculations.

_____ 6. Jars and syringes are the only packages that do not have childproof caps or lids.

_____ 7. All records are to be kept in the pharmacy for only 1 year from the time the medication was prepared.

_____ 8. The recordkeeping part of compounding is extremely important.

_____ 9. Capsule size 000 is the smallest size.

_____ 10. Graduated cylinders are available in both conical and cylindrical shapes.

## MULTIPLE CHOICE

Complete each question by circling the best answer.

1. Which of the following is *not* a reason the pharmacy repackages a bulk drug into unit-dose?
   A. The cost is lower when this process is done by the hospital
   B. Manufacturers do not package the drug in unit-dose
   C. Unit-dose medications can be recycled and used on another patient
   D. Unit-dose is easier to count

2. The dosage form normally repackaged in a pharmacy is the
   A. Tablet form
   B. Capsule form
   C. Liquid form
   D. All of the above

3. The expiration date on a drug is 2/07; the drug expires on
   A. The first day of February 2007
   B. The last day of February 2007
   C. The first day of July 2002
   D. The last day of July 2002

4. The most common nonsterile, compounded items in a hospital are
   A. Creams, ointments, and oral suspensions
   B. Tablets, capsules, and liquids
   C. All of the above
   D. None of the above

5. A factor that can affect the stability of a drug is
   A. Light
   B. Air
   C. Temperature
   D. All of the above

6. The punch method is used to prepare
   A. Solutions
   B. Tablets
   C. Capsules
   D. Ointments

7. Good manufacturing practices do not include which of the following?
   A. Equipment in good and clean condition
   B. Medications checked by a technician
   C. Appropriate packaging for the drugs
   D. Records logged for referencing

8. A class _____ balance weighs _____ substances, and a class _____ balance weighs _____ substances.
   A. A, lighter; B, heavier
   B. A, heavier; B, lighter
   C. A, both heavy and light; B, both heavy and light

Copyright © 2007 Elsevier, Inc. All rights reserved.

## MATCHING

**Matching I**

_____ 1. Unit-dose

_____ 2. Monthly supply

_____ 3. Recipe book

_____ 4. Dosage form

_____ 5. Mortar and pestle

A. Tablet, capsule, spansule

B. One medication dose per container

C. Compounding equipment

D. 30-Day supply

E. Formula cards

**Matching II**

Match the following dosage forms with their auxiliary labels.

_____ 1. Ophthalmics

_____ 2. Otics

_____ 3. Ointments, creams, lotions

_____ 4. Suppositories

_____ 5. Patches

A. For topical use; external use

B. Apply to skin

C. For rectal use

D. For the eye

E. For the ear

## FILL IN THE BLANK

1. What auxiliary label is used with suspensions? _____

2. The base ingredient of a suppository is usually a combination of _____ and _____.

3. You must have liquids at _____ level to read the bottom of the liquid line, known as the _____.

4. To prepare an ointment, a _____ base must be mixed with the drug. To prepare a cream, a _____ base is used.

5. What type of compounding equipment is used to weigh powders? _____

6. A _____ and _____ are used to crush tablets and other solid substances.

7. Name three additional ingredients used to reduce the bad taste of drugs.

   A. _____

   B. _____

   C. _____

## SHORT ANSWER

1. Why is it necessary to use tweezers to grasp metal weights?

_____

_____

## RESEARCH ACTIVITY

Access the following compounding websites:
_www.pccarx.com_
_www.pharmacytimes.com/compounding_

1. What kind of services do they provide?

Copyright © 2007 Elsevier, Inc. All rights reserved.

2. Find an interesting recipe (if published). Print it and share it with the class.

3. Is membership required to use these sites and to obtain their products?

## CRITICAL THINKING

1. Pediatric medications sometimes require special compounding. What are some ways the pharmacy staff can accommodate pediatric patients to foster their compliance in taking their medications?

2. Preparing capsules using the punch method can be messy. What techniques for preparing capsules can you develop to minimize the mess?

3. Mrs. Foster has been coming to your pharmacy for years. Lately she has become hard of hearing and often misinterprets the pharmacist's directions about her medications.
   A. How can you, as a technician, aid in this process?
   B. What tools can you develop to better help Mrs. Foster understand how to take her medications?

Copyright © 2007 Elsevier, Inc. All rights reserved.

# 13 Aseptic Technique

## TERMS AND DEFINITIONS

Select the correct term from the following list and write the corresponding letter in the blank next to the statement.

A. Aseptic technique

B. Gauge

C. Horizontal flow hood

D. Hyperalimentation

E. Laminar flow hood

F. Parenterals

G. Peripheral parenterals

H. Total parenteral nutrition

I. Universal precautions

J. Vertical flow hood

_____ 1. The size of the needle opening

_____ 2. Environment for preparation of sterile products within a streamline flow near a solid boundary

_____ 3. Parenteral nutrition for individuals unable to eat

_____ 4. A set of standards used in the preparation of medications that reduces the chance of contamination

_____ 5. Medications administered by injection, such as intravenously or intramuscularly; introduced in a manner other than by way of the intestines

_____ 6. The procedure used to eliminate the possibility of a drug becoming contaminated with microbes or particles

_____ 7. Large-volume IV nutrition administered through the central vein, which allows for a higher concentration of solutions

_____ 8. Environment for preparation of sterile products that uses air originating from the back of the hood moving forward across the hood out into the room

_____ 9. Injection of a medication into the veins on the periphery of the body instead of into a central vein or artery

_____ 10. Environment for preparation of chemotherapy treatments that uses air originating from the roof of the hood moving downward and captured in a vent on the floor of the hood

## TRUE OR FALSE

Write T or F next to each statement.

_____ 1. One of the most trivial responsibilities a hospital pharmacy technician can have is the proper preparation of parenteral medications.

_____ 2. All parenteral and ophthalmic medications should be prepared within a laminar flow hood.

_____ 3. Cost can be a determining factor in the choice of some pharmacy equipment.

_____ 4. All syringes must have a transfer needle if transported out of the pharmacy.

_____ 5. Flexible bags and bottles are the main types of piggyback containers.

_____ 6. Most syringes are made of glass and are meant to be sterilized and reused.

_____ 7. The purpose of needles in pharmacy is to draw solution up into the syringe.

_____ 8. To ensure sterility, the needle shaft must be wiped with alcohol.

Copyright © 2007 Elsevier, Inc. All rights reserved.

_____ 9. All chemotherapeutic agents should be prepared in a vertical flow hood.

_____ 10. All IV rooms have reference books that can be used to find special instructions for all types of parenteral medications.

## MULTIPLE CHOICE

Complete each question by circling the best answer.

1. An *MDV* is a
   A. Multiple drug vehicle
   B. Multiple dose vial
   C. Metered dose ventilator
   D. None of the above

2. Which of the following is *not* a parenteral route of administration?
   A. IV
   B. IM
   C. SL
   D. SQ

3. Insulin must be put only into
   A. Glass containers
   B. Small-volume drips
   C. Syringe pumps
   D. Viaflex bags

4. Which of the following is *not* an example of a medication administration system?
   A. IV chamber
   B. CRIS
   C. CAD pump
   D. None of the above

5. A chunk of rubber is dislodged and falls into the vial; this is called
   A. Filtering
   B. Beveling
   C. Coring
   D. Piggybacking

6. To ensure sterility, what part of the needle should not be touched?
   A. Hub
   B. Shaft
   C. Bevel
   D. All of the above

7. When aseptic technique is used, what should not be worn?
   A. Gloves
   B. Artificial nails
   C. Hair ties
   D. All of the above

8. For proper handwashing technique, you should wash which areas for 30 to 90 seconds?
   A. Hands, face, and arms
   B. Hands, wrists, and arms
   C. Fingernails, wrists, and underarms
   D. Fingernails, hands, and face

9. To clean the hood you should use
   A. Soap and water
   B. Antimicrobial soap and hot water
   C. 70% Isopropyl alcohol
   D. Hydrogen peroxide

10. The Julian Date is
    A. The actual consecutive day of the year
    B. Julian's birthday
    C. January 1
    D. December 31

## FILL IN THE BLANK

1. All parenteral medications should be prepared in a manner that reduces the possibility of _____.

2. Large-volume drips include three sizes: _____, _____, and _____.

3. Microdrip chambers are most often used for _____ patients.

4. A _____ is a preset amount of drug that can be administered by the patient when pain intensifies.

5. Two types of syringes commercially available are _____ and _____.

6. The rule to remember when sizing needles is that the gauge (size) number of the needle is _____ to the needle's bore size.

7. The smallest size filter is the _____ filter.

8. Aseptic technique goes hand-in-hand with _____ _____.

9. All work done in the hood is to be done _____ within the hood.

10. What type of filter is used in the hood to trap all particles larger than 0.2 μm? _____

Copyright © 2007 Elsevier, Inc. All rights reserved.

## EXPLAIN

1. What is the process for breaking an ampule? _____
_____

2. How are chemotherapy wastes disposed of? _____
_____

3. Why are dextrose, amino acids, and lipids used in TPNs?
_____
_____
_____

4. Why are syringes not reused when a change is made from one drug to another?
_____
_____

5. Why is the placement of the hands so important when sterile products are prepared? _____
_____

## SHORT ANSWER

1. Name two types of hyperalimentation: _____ and _____

2. When preparing chemotherapy agents, you must wear _____ and _____.

3. Needles are made either of _____ or _____.

4. The _____ route is the most dangerous to the patient because it bypasses the body's most _____ barriers and directly enters the _____.

5. A _____ _____ is used to draw up medications from an _____.

## RESEARCH ACTIVITY

Access the websites *www.usp797.org* and *www.globalrph.com/aseptic.htm.*

1. What is USP 797 all about?

2. Read through all the information presented on aseptic technique.

3. Take note of the precautions for patient care.

Copyright © 2007 Elsevier, Inc. All rights reserved.

1. You have been preparing injections in the IV room and suddenly stick your finger with a needle. What went wrong? What mistake did you make that caused you to stick your finger?

2. If you stick your finger with a sterile needle, is it necessary to go to the emergency department for treatment?

3. You have been assigned to work in the IV preparation room for your shift. What are the first items you need to take care of when you walk into the IV room? What aseptic technique requirements need to be followed before you begin preparation of IVs?

4. What should you do at the end of your shift to ensure a smooth workflow when your replacement technician comes to relieve you?

Copyright © 2007 Elsevier, Inc. All rights reserved.

# 14 Pharmacy Stock and Billing

## TERMS AND DEFINITIONS

Select the correct term from the following list and write the corresponding letter in the blank next to the statement.

A. Adjudication

B. Formulary

C. Generic name

D. POS

E. Recall

F. Trade name

_____ 1. Nonproprietary name of a drug

_____ 2. Required return of a drug or device to the manufacturer because of failure to meet FDA standards

_____ 3. Electronic insurance billing for medication payment

_____ 4. Point of sale

_____ 5. Brand name of a drug

_____ 6. A list of approved drugs to be stocked by the pharmacy; also, a list of drugs covered by an insurance company

## TRUE OR FALSE

Write T or F next to each statement.

_____ 1. A pharmacy technician often is put in charge of billing.

_____ 2. A formulary is a book that contains compounding recipes.

_____ 3. Most formulary drugs are generic drugs.

_____ 4. Generic drugs are less expensive because they are less effective than brand name drugs.

_____ 5. In a PPO, the patient must select a physician from the insurance plan's list.

_____ 6. A PPO plan usually has a higher copayment than an HMO.

_____ 7. If an insurance claim is rejected, the technician must call the help desk to find out why.

_____ 8. Each insurance plan has specific guidelines that must be followed for reimbursement to be made.

_____ 9. The cost of prescriptions is the same from pharmacy to pharmacy.

_____ 10. A patient may call for a refill after 1 week from the day the person filled the prescription, as long as there are refills remaining.

_____ 11. If the cardholder's information does not match up to the processor's information, the patient does not have coverage.

_____ 12. Automated systems are switching over from entering personal identifying codes to using fingerprint ID only.

_____ 13. One of the best ways to learn drug names and to become familiar with the drugs' location in your pharmacy is to put away new stock.

_____ 14. Recall notices arrive by voice mail.

_____ 15. Cytotoxic drugs do not need special paperwork when they are returned to the manufacturer.

## MULTIPLE CHOICE

Complete the question by circling the best answer.

1. Who is responsible for maintaining the inventory stock in the pharmacy?
   A. Pharmacist
   B. Technician
   C. Inventory technician
   D. All of the above

2. The types of drugs included in a formulary are
   A. New drugs
   B. Generic drugs
   C. Uncommon drugs
   D. Extremely expensive drugs

**55**

Copyright © 2007 Elsevier, Inc. All rights reserved.

3. In third-party billing, the third party is the
   A. Pharmacy
   B. Patient
   C. Insurance company
   D. All of the above

4. Which of the following is *not* a type of insurance plan in use today?
   A. POS
   B. HMO
   C. PPO
   D. Medicare

5. Which of the following is *not* a special feature of an HMO?
   A. Primary care physician
   B. Independent physician's association
   C. Copayment
   D. Workers' compensation

6. Which of the following is *not* a difference between HMOs and PPOs?
   A. A PPO plan has no requirements for a PCP
   B. PPO plans have a copayment
   C. PPO plans have a deductible
   D. All of the above

7. The amount a patient must pay before the copay starts is called the
   A. Share of cost
   B. Penalty period
   C. Deductible
   D. Grace period

8. Which of the following is *not* a government-run insurance program?
   A. Medicare
   B. Medicaid
   C. Long-term disability
   D. Worker's compensation

9. Which group is *not* covered by Medicare?
   A. Infant patients
   B. Disabled patients
   C. Senior patients
   D. Dialysis patients

10. The insurance company decides the amount of coverage per medication based on
    A. AWP
    B. Copay

C. DAW
D. A and B

11. Which of the following is *not* a reason for the insurance company to reject a claim?
    A. Coverage has expired
    B. Use of a generic drug
    C. Refill too soon
    D. NDC not covered

12. Some patients are exempt from insurance limitations because of their illness or disease. Which group of patients is *not* exempt?
    A. Diabetic patients
    B. Cancer patients
    C. HIV patients
    D. AIDS patients

13. Sometimes insurance companies refill medications early because
    A. The patient lost the medication
    B. The patient is going on a vacation
    C. The physician told the patient to increase the dosage
    D. A and C

14. Which of the following is *not* an example of an inventory system that can keep a running inventory of medications, as well as order them?
    A. SOC system
    B. POS system
    C. Order card system
    D. Hand-held inventory computer system

15. Which of the following is *not* a reason to return medications to the warehouse or manufacturer?
    A. Drug recalled
    B. Drug damaged during delivery
    C. Drug incorrectly reconstituted
    D. Drug expired

16. Manufacturers are required by law to recall any product that has been found to have which of the following guideline violations?
    A. Labeling is wrong
    B. Product was not packaged or produced properly
    C. Drug batch was contaminated
    D. All of the above

## FILL IN THE BLANK

1. An HMO is an effective method of controlling _____.

2. An HMO may require _____ authorization (PA) on certain medications.

3. The difference between HMOs and PPOs is that the patient usually pays more _____ expenses for PPOs.

4. Each state has its own _____ program for low-income residents.

5. The required information that insurance companies must have to process a claim from the pharmacy or to reimburse a patient is the same as on a _____.

Copyright © 2007 Elsevier, Inc. All rights reserved.

6. _____ _____ is a type of insurance paid by _____ to fully cover injuries suffered by _____ while on the job.

## SHORT ANSWER

1. When billing an insurance company for medication, what is the minimum information the insurance company requires?

_____

_____

2. One of the most common problems resulting in a claim rejection is a non-ID match. What patient information should be double-checked in these cases?

_____

_____

3. Why do many pharmacies have a policy of pulling off the shelves any medication that will expire in 3 months or sooner?

_____

_____

4. What are the three main responsibilities of automated return companies?

A. _____

B. _____

C. _____

5. To what categories of drugs must the pharmacy give special consideration? Why?

_____

_____

## EXPLAIN

1. What are the three Medicare levels available?

A. Medicare Part A _____

B. Medicare Part B _____

C. Medicare Part D _____

2. What are the three types of Medicare Part D plans, as outlined by *Consumer Reports?*

_____

_____

_____

## RESEARCH ACTIVITY

1. Access the website *www.fda.gov.→FDA news→recalls, product safety*
   A. Find three drugs that have been recalled.
   B. What were the reasons for the recalls?

Copyright © 2007 Elsevier, Inc. All rights reserved.

2. Make a phone call or speak to someone who has an HMO, PPO health insurance policy.
   A. What is their drug coverage?
   B. Is there a copay for generic/brand drugs?

## CRITICAL THINKING

1. Should Medicare cover all medical and prescriptions costs for elderly patients? Give three pros and three cons for this issue.

2. Many Canadian pharmacies are offering prescription drugs at vastly reduced prices compared with U.S. prices. Is there any reason not to "go across the border" for your medications?

3. Choosing an insurance health plan can be overwhelming. What type of coverage would best meet your needs? Outline all items you would need to have total health coverage.

Copyright © 2007 Elsevier, Inc. All rights reserved.

# 15 Psychopharmacology

## TERMS AND DEFINITIONS

Select the correct term from the following list and write the corresponding letter in the blank next to the statement.

A. Anxiety

B. Bipolar disorder

C. Depression

D. Dystonia

E. Extrapyramidal

F. Insomnia

G. Mania

H. Neurosis

I. Pruritus

J. Psychosis

K. Schizophrenia

L. Tardive dyskinesia

M. Tourette's syndrome

_____ 1. Symptoms that include twisting, repeated jerking movements, and/or abnormal posture

_____ 2. Symptoms indicating that a patient is taking antipsychotic medications, including parkinsonism, dystonias, and tremors

_____ 3. Severe itching that can be caused by an allergic reaction

_____ 4. Depressive psychosis, alternating between excessive phases of mania and depression; formerly known as manic-depressive

_____ 5. A form of psychosis characterized by excessive excitement, elevated moods, and exalted feelings

_____ 6. A disorder characterized by multiple motor tics, lack of muscle coordination, and involuntary, purposeless movements accompanied by grunts and barks

_____ 7. Feelings of apprehension, dread, and fear, with characteristics including tension, restlessness, tachycardia, dyspnea, and a sense of hopelessness

_____ 8. A mental state characterized by sadness, a feeling of loss, grief, loss of appetite, and possibly suicidal thoughts

_____ 9. A mental illness characterized by loss of contact with reality

_____ 10. Unwanted side effects of treatment with phenothiazines, including slow, rhythmical, involuntary movements that are either generalized or specific to a muscle group

_____ 11. A group of mental disorders characterized by inappropriate emotions and unrealistic thinking

_____ 12. Mental illness, without loss of contact with reality, arising from stress or anxiety factors in the patient's environment; phobias can be listed in this category

_____ 13. Difficulty falling or staying asleep

Copyright © 2007 Elsevier, Inc. All rights reserved.

## TRUE OR FALSE

Write T or F next to each statement.

____ 1. Because of the brain's complexity, the study of the brain is one of the most difficult disciplines in medicine.

____ 2. Psychologists can write prescriptions for mental health.

____ 3. The nervous system is an intricate network of bones and muscles.

____ 4. Because of the wide range of mental conditions, many alternative treatments are available.

____ 5. Everyone suffers from depression at some time.

____ 6. Patients with bipolar disorder are commonly called *manic-depressives.*

____ 7. TCAs, MAOIs, and SSRIs, when taken for depression, may be taken concurrently.

____ 8. A major cause of insomnia is stress.

____ 9. The use of barbiturates and benzodiazepines is a good and permanent solution for long-term insomnia.

____ 10. Antipsychotic medications are effective at reducing nausea and vomiting.

## MULTIPLE CHOICE

Complete each question by circling the best answer.

1. Which of the following is *not* an antipsychotic agent?
   A. Haldol
   B. Desyrel
   C. Orap
   D. Zyprexa

2. Traditionally, mentally ill patients were treated with
   A. Electrical shock
   B. Straightjackets
   C. Isolation
   D. A, B, and C

3. The field of psychology is the study of
   A. Human behavior
   B. Human emotions
   C. Human behavior and emotions
   D. Human emotions, feelings, and behavior

4. Which of the following is *not* a specialist in the field of mental health?
   A. Psychiatrist
   B. Counselor
   C. Bartender
   D. Psychologist

5. Which of the following is *not* an example of group therapy?
   A. Confessional
   B. Alcoholics Anonymous
   C. Weight Watchers
   D. Narcotics Anonymous

6. Which mental health specialist(s) can write prescriptions?
   A. Psychologist
   B. Psychiatrist
   C. Neurologist
   D. B and C

7. Schizophrenia, mania, and psychotic depression can be treated with
   A. Antipsychotics
   B. Antidepressants
   C. Tranquilizers
   D. All of the above

8. Elavil, Pamelor, and Tofranil are all examples of
   A. Antipsychotics
   B. Antidepressants
   C. Antianxiety agents
   D. Insomnia agents

9. Which class of antidepressants can be prescribed for chronic pain?
   A. TCAs
   B. MAOIs
   C. SSRIs
   D. OTCs

10. Which class of drug interacts with many foods and OTC agents?
    A. TCAs
    B. MAOIs
    C. SSRIs
    D. MOAs

11. Paxil, Prozac, and Zoloft are all examples of
    A. TCAs
    B. MAOIs
    C. SSRIs
    D. OTCs

12. Which two types of drugs must not be taken together?
    A. TCAs and MAOIs
    B. TCAs and SSRIs
    C. MAOIs and SSRIs
    D. None of the above

Copyright © 2007 Elsevier, Inc. All rights reserved.

13. The drug bupropion is also indicated for
    A. Weight loss
    B. Smoking cessation
    C. Alcohol withdrawal
    D. Hiccup relief

14. Antipsychotics, antidepressants, antianxiety drugs, and benzodiazepines should all have which auxiliary label?
    A. Take at bedtime
    B. Take with food
    C. Avoid dairy products
    D. May cause drowsiness and dizziness

15. Imipramine is indicated for enuresis, which is
    A. An eating disorder
    B. Insomnia
    C. Bedwetting
    D. Loss of hair

16. The most common ingredient in OTC sleep aids is
    A. Diphenhydrinate
    B. Diphenhydramine
    C. Acetaminophen
    D. Digoxin

## FILL IN THE BLANK

1. The two main classifications of antipsychotic drugs are _____ and _____, and their mechanism of action is the inhibition of _____ in the CNS.

2. _____ is used to treat the mania phase of bipolar disorder.

3. What are the three closely related agents used to treat depression?

    A. _____

    B. _____

    C. _____

4. Antidepressants increase the _____, _____, and _____ chemicals in the brain.

5. Two classes of drugs used for short-term treatment of insomnia are _____ and _____; these drugs act on different parts of the brain.

6. The main use of hypnotics is to _____ _____.

7. Antianxiety agents affect the CNS, producing _____ effects.

8. What are two side effects of antipsychotic agents?

    A. _____

    B. _____

9. MAOIs react with foods containing _____, which can cause a hypertensive _____.

10. The brain is protected by the _____ _____ _____, which prevents many _____ from passing into it.

## MATCHING

### Matching I
Match the drug classifications with their indications.

____ 1. Antipsychotic agents    A. Induce sleep

____ 2. Hypnotics    B. Preferable treatment for depression and OCD

____ 3. MAOIs    C. Used to relax and ease a nervous or irritated person

____ 4. SSRIs    D. Treats psychosis, nausea, and vomiting

____ 5. Sedatives    E. Can cause hypertension

### Matching II
Match the drugs with their classifications.

____ 1. Haldol    A. Sedative (barbiturate)

____ 2. Celexa    B. Antianxiety agent

____ 3. Phenobarbital    C. Antipsychotic

____ 4. Xanax    D. Hypnotic

____ 5. Ambien    E. SSRI antidepressant

Copyright © 2007 Elsevier, Inc. All rights reserved.

**Matching III**

Match the following trade and generic drug names.

____ 1. Valium       A. Amitriptyline

____ 2. Zoloft       B. Risperidone

____ 3. Elavil       C. Diazepam

____ 4. Risperdal       D. Prochlorperazine

____ 5. Compazine       E. Sertraline

## RESEARCH ACTIVITY

1. Access the website *http://en.wikipedia.org/wiki/psychopharmacology*
   A. Read the history section.
   B. What is the connection between opioids and psychotropic drugs?

2. Access the website *www.nida.nih.gov/infofacts/Ritalin.html*
   A. How does Ritalin work?
   B. What neurotransmitter in the brain does it affect?
   C. Is it really effective against ADHD?

## CRITICAL THINKING

1. Give three reasons so many people are becoming addicted to prescription drugs.

2. What is contributing to the rise in ADD/ADHD/OCD in children? Does it have anything to do with preservatives or hormones in food?

3. When a person is categorized as "neurotic" and a "hypochondriac," what exactly does this mean? Do you think there is any "cure" for those conditions? Are they real psychological conditions that can be treated?

Copyright © 2007 Elsevier, Inc. All rights reserved.

# 16 Endocrine System

## TERMS AND DEFINITIONS

Select the correct term from the following list and write the corresponding letter in the blank next to the statement.

A. Addison's disease

B. Autoimmune disease

C. Cretinism

D. Cushing's disease

E. Euthyroid

F. Exophthalmos

G. Glucose

H. Goiter

I. Graves' disease

J. Hormones

K. Hypercalcemia

L. Hypocalcemia

M. Hyperglycemia

N. Hypoglycemia

O. Myxedema

P. Osteoporosis

Q. Paget's disease

R. Thyroxine

S. Triiodothyronine

_____ 1. Condition in which the development of the brain and body is inhibited by a congenital lack of thyroid secretion

_____ 2. Condition that affects older adults in which the density of the bones decreases, resulting in softening and weakening

_____ 3. Prominence of the eyeball caused by increased thyroid hormone

_____ 4. Abnormally low glucose content circulating in the bloodstream

_____ 5. Condition caused by hypersecretion of thyroid with diffuse goiter, exophthalmos, and skin changes

_____ 6. Unusually high concentration of calcium in the blood

_____ 7. Normally functioning thyroid gland

_____ 8. Simple sugar

_____ 9. Condition resulting in a decrease in adrenocortical hormones, such as mineralocorticoids and glucocorticoids, and the appearance of symptoms such as muscle weakness and weight loss

_____ 10. Low concentration of calcium in the blood

_____ 11. Condition associated with a decrease in bone mass and softening of the bones, resulting in a greater possibility of bone fractures

_____ 12. Known as $T_3$; contains three ions of iodine

_____ 13. Abnormally high glucose content circulating in the bloodstream

_____ 14. Syndrome that causes increased secretion by the adrenal cortex with excessive production of glucocorticoids, resulting in symptoms such as a moon face and deposits of fat (buffalo hump)

_____ 15. Chemical substances produced and secreted by an endocrine duct into the bloodstream or into another duct, resulting in a physiologic response at a specific target tissue

_____ 16. Condition in which a person's tissues are attacked by the person's own immune system; abnormal antigen-antibody reaction

_____ 17. Condition associated with a decrease in overall thyroid function in adults; also known as hypothyroidism

Copyright © 2007 Elsevier, Inc. All rights reserved.

_____ 18. Condition in which the thyroid is enlarged because of a lack of iodine; known as a simple goiter or, if a tumor is the cause, as a toxic goiter

_____ 19. Known as $T_4$; contains four iodine ions

## TRUE OR FALSE

Write T or F next to each statement.

_____ 1. The Greek word for hormone means "to excite."

_____ 2. Hormones control women and their moods only.

_____ 3. All hormones are composed of proteins.

_____ 4. Steroids enter and attach to receptor sites inside the cell.

_____ 5. Melatonin is a chemical substance that helps control the skin's ability to tan.

_____ 6. The pituitary gland is referred to as the *master gland.*

_____ 7. Calcium is the major mineral found in bones.

_____ 8. The pancreas is not the largest organ of the endocrine system.

_____ 9. Men stop producing sperm at some point during their midlife crisis.

_____ 10. The most well-known condition that can affect the pancreas is diabetes.

## SYSTEM IDENTIFIER

Identify each organ in this system and enter the term next to the corresponding number.

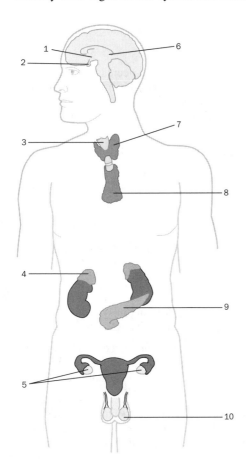

1. _____

2. _____

3. _____

4. _____

5. _____

6. _____

7. _____

8. _____

9. _____

10. _____

Copyright © 2007 Elsevier, Inc. All rights reserved.

## MULTIPLE CHOICE

Complete each question by circling the best answer.

1. PTU and methimazole are used for the treatment of
   A. Diabetes
   B. Osteoporosis
   C. Hyperthyroidism
   D. Estrogen replacement

2. Fosamax and Calcimar are used for the treatment of
   A. Diabetes
   B. Osteoporosis
   C. Hyperthyroidism
   D. Estrogen replacement

3. The gland that secretes hormones that help the body keep calcium levels adequate is the
   A. Thyroid
   B. Parathyroid
   C. Hypothalamus
   D. Pituitary

4. The largest endocrine gland is the _____, which produces insulin and glucagon
   A. Thyroid
   B. Pituitary
   C. Thymus
   D. Pancreas

5. Which of the following is *not* a system that influences the endocrine system?
   A. Positive feedback
   B. Hormonal chemicals that participate in a chain reaction
   C. Negative feedback
   D. Nervous system

6. Which gland influences water balance, body temperature, appetite, and emotions?
   A. Pancreas
   B. Thymus
   C. Thyroid
   D. Hypothalamus

7. Which glands participate in the activities of the kidneys?
   A. Adrenals
   B. Ovaries
   C. Testes
   D. None of the above

8. Failure of the endocrine system to perform correctly affects what area of the body?
   A. Heart
   B. Kidney
   C. Brain
   D. All of the above

9. A goiter is an enlargement of the
   A. Prostate gland
   B. Pituitary gland
   C. Thyroid gland
   D. Testes

10. Aplasia affects children born without a
    A. Pineal gland
    B. Pituitary gland
    C. Thyroid gland
    D. Pancreas

11. Conditions such as abnormal uterine bleeding, post-menopausal osteoporosis, and advanced prostatic carcinomas can be treated with
    A. Estrogen
    B. Progesterone
    C. Testosterone
    D. Insulin

12. Conditions such as breast carcinomas in women, certain types of anemia, and androgen deficiency can be treated with
    A. Estrogen
    B. Progesterone
    C. Testosterone
    D. Insulin

## FILL IN THE BLANK

1. The _____, _____, and _____ glands, located in the brain, play an important role in hormone production.

2. The _____ is the bridge between the nervous system and the hormone system.

3. _____ hormones act on the cell from which they were secreted, and _____ hormones act on cells near target cells.

4. Two mechanisms of action of glands are _____ and _____.

5. The two different types of hormones in the endocrine systems are _____ and _____.

6. The two hormones involved in the "fight or flight reaction" are _____ and _____.

7. The ovaries produce the hormones _____ and _____, and the testes produce _____.

Copyright © 2007 Elsevier, Inc. All rights reserved.

8. The hormone _____ is responsible for the beginning stages of labor.

9. _____, _____, and _____ are three types of steroids produced in the adrenal cortex.

10. The cause of insulin-dependent diabetes mellitus is the inability of the _____ to produce _____.

## MATCHING

**Matching I**
Match the drugs with their indications.

_____ 1. Synthroid      A. Addison's disease

_____ 2. Glucophage      B. Inflammation

_____ 3. Florinef      C. Thyroid replacement

_____ 4. Prednisone      D. Hypercalcemia

_____ 5. Aredia      E. Oral antidiabetic

**Matching II**
Match the trade and generic drug names.

_____ 1. Synthroid      A. alendronate

_____ 2. Fosamax      B. conjugated estrogens

_____ 3. Florinef      C. pioglitazone

_____ 4. Premarin      D. levothyroxine

_____ 5. Actos      E. fludrocortisone acetate

## RESEARCH ACTIVITY

1. Access the website *www.nida.nih.gov/infofacts/steroids*. Find information on anabolic steroids that would enable you to answer the following questions:
   A. What are they?
   B. Who uses them and why?
   C. What are the side effects?
   D. In what controlled substance category are they included?

2. Go to *www.nof.org/osteoporosis/index*. Find out the answers to the following questions:
   A. What is osteoporosis?
   B. The lack of what hormone is a contributing factor?
   C. What are some solutions for osteoporosis?

## CRITICAL THINKING

1. Diabetes mellitus has been prevalent in your family for the past few years. What lifestyle changes should you make to avoid being diagnosed with this disease?

2. When a young person goes through the adolescence stage of development, the pituitary gland releases hormones that bring about many physical and emotional changes. How many hormones are released, and what parts of the body are affected? What emotional changes take place?

3. The hormone content of meat has been the subject of numerous discussions. Do hormones in meat really affect us physically? If so, how?

Copyright © 2007 Elsevier, Inc. All rights reserved.

# 17 Nervous System

## TERMS AND DEFINITIONS

Select the correct term from the following list and write the corresponding letter in the blank next to the statement.

A. Afferent

B. Autonomic

C. Axon

D. Blood-brain barrier

E. Cell body

F. Cerebrospinal fluid (CSF)

G. Cervical

H. Dendrites

I. Efferent

J. Homeostasis

K. Lumbar

L. Monoamine oxidase (MAO)

M. Nerve terminal

N. Neuron

O. Parasympathetic nervous system

P. Peripheral nervous system

Q. Somatic

R. Sympathetic nervous system

S. Thoracic

_____ 1. The motor neurons that control voluntary actions of the skeletal muscles

_____ 2. The main part of a neuron from which axons and dendrites extend

_____ 3. An enzyme (includes MAO-A and MAO-B) found in the nerve terminals and liver cells; inactivates chemicals such as tyramine, catecholamines, serotonin, and certain medications

_____ 4. The segment of a neuron that branches out to bring impulses to the cell body

_____ 5. The conduction of electrical impulses away from the central nervous system to the body

_____ 6. The part of a nerve cell that conducts impulses away from the cell body

_____ 7. The region of the back that includes the area between the ribs and the pelvis; the area around the waist

_____ 8. Division of the autonomic nervous system that functions during restful situations; the "breed or feed" part of the ANS

_____ 9. The equilibrium pertaining to the balance in the body of fluids, pH level, and chemicals

_____ 10. Relates to the area of the thorax or the chest

_____ 11. A fluid that fills the ventricles of the brain and also lies in the space between the arachnoid layer of the meninges, brain, or spinal cord

_____ 12. The functional unit of the nervous system that includes the cell body, dendrites, axons, and terminals

_____ 13. The end portion of the neuron where nerve impulses cause chemicals to be released; these cross a small space, called a *synaptic cleft*, to carry the impulse to another neuron

_____ 14. Division of the autonomic nervous system that functions during stressful situations; the "flight or fight" part of the ANS

_____ 15. Self-controlling or involuntary

_____ 16. Division of the nervous system outside the brain and spinal cord

_____ 17. A barrier formed by special characteristics of capillaries that prevents certain chemicals from moving into the brain

_____ 18. The direction of neuronal impulses from the body toward the central nervous system

_____ 19. The neck region

**67**

Copyright © 2007 Elsevier, Inc. All rights reserved.

## TRUE OR FALSE

Write T or F next to each statement.

_____ 1. The human nervous system is a simple body system.

_____ 2. The central nervous system consists of the brain and spinal cord.

_____ 3. The nerve impulses are transmitted by various chemicals, called *neurotransmitters*.

_____ 4. Most drugs that can pass through the blood-brain barrier are water soluble.

_____ 5. The somatic nervous system is part of the CNS.

_____ 6. The sympathetic and parasympathetic systems are part of the autonomic nervous system.

_____ 7. Individuals with Parkinson's disease have low levels of dopamine.

_____ 8. Few differences can be found between the sympathetic and parasympathetic systems.

_____ 9. Skeletal muscle relaxants are not meant for long-term use.

_____ 10. Patients with epilepsy need to take their medication only after a seizure.

## MULTIPLE CHOICE

Complete each question by circling the best answer.

1. The smallest functional part of the central nervous system is the
   A. Brain
   B. Synapse
   C. Spinal cord
   D. Neuron

2. The largest area of the brain is the
   A. Cerebrum
   B. Cerebellum
   C. Thalamus
   D. Hypothalamus

3. The midbrain, pons, and medulla oblongata are all part of the
   A. Cerebrum
   B. Brainstem
   C. Cerebellum
   D. Spinal cord

4. Which of the following is *not* a main neurotransmitter of the sympathetic system?
   A. Dopamine
   B. Epinephrine
   C. Acetylcholine
   D. Norepinephrine

5. A patient suffering from premature labor could be given
   A. Levophed
   B. Intropin
   C. Yutopar
   D. Pitocin

6. Dry mouth and inhibition of urine output are side effects of
   A. Sympathomimetics
   B. Anticholinergics
   C. Adrenergics
   D. Parasympathomimetics

7. Which of the following is not a generalized seizure?
   A. Petit mal
   B. Status epilepticus
   C. Tonic-clonic
   D. None of the above

8. Besides taking their medications, individuals with epilepsy can help themselves by
   A. Learning relaxation techniques
   B. Avoiding flashing lights
   C. A and B
   D. None of the above

9. An abnormal loss of memory and basic mental function is called
   A. Epilepsy
   B. Dementia
   C. Seizures
   D. Blood-brain barrier

10. A condition associated with loss or a deficiency of dopamine is
    A. Alzheimer's disease
    B. Parkinson's disease
    C. Multiple sclerosis
    D. Lou Gehrig's disease

Copyright © 2007 Elsevier, Inc. All rights reserved.

## FILL IN THE BLANK

1. The three main states of a neuron are _____, _____, and _____.

2. The hypothalamus is a _____ and _____.

3. The thin covering that protects the brain and spinal cord from the bony structures of the skull and spinal column is the _____.

4. The two branches of the PNS are called the _____ and _____ nervous systems, which regulate _____ and _____.

5. Drugs that mimic the actions of the sympathetic nervous system are called _____ and drugs that mimic the parasympathetic nervous system are called _____.

6. Alpha receptors are located on _____; beta$_1$-receptors are located on the _____, and beta$_2$-receptors are located in the _____ and elsewhere.

7. The function of the sympathetic division is to respond to _____ situations; one of the main functions of the parasympathetic system is to activate the _____ system.

8. The main neurotransmitters of the sympathetic system are _____ and _____, and the main neurotransmitter of the parasympathetic system is _____.

9. The two main types of skeletal muscle relaxants are _____ acting and _____ acting.

10. The main class of drugs used to treat myasthenia gravis is _____.

## MATCHING

### Matching I

Match the following disease states with their drug treatment classes.

| | |
|---|---|
| _____ 1. Epilepsy | A. Autoimmune stimulants (interferons) |
| _____ 2. Alzheimer's disease | B. Dopamine-increasing drugs |
| _____ 3. Multiple sclerosis | C. Cholinesterase inhibitors |
| _____ 4. Parkinson's disease | D. Riluzole |
| _____ 5. ALS | E. Anticonvulsants |

### Matching II

Match the following drugs with the diseases they treat.

| | |
|---|---|
| _____ 1. Phenytoin | A. Parkinson's disease |
| _____ 2. Aricept | B. Myasthenia gravis |
| _____ 3. Dantrium | C. Alzheimer's disease |
| _____ 4. Sinemet | D. Epilepsy |
| _____ 5. Mestinon | E. Multiple sclerosis |

## SHORT ANSWER

1. What are the most common symptoms of Parkinson's disease? _____, _____, _____, _____, _____

2. What happens to the brain cells in a patient with Alzheimer's disease? _____

_____

_____

3. Name four drug therapies used in the treatment of seizures: _____, _____, _____, _____

**69**

Copyright © 2007 Elsevier, Inc. All rights reserved.

1. Access the website *http://en.wikipedia.org/wiki/caffeine* and answer the following questions:
   A   Where is caffeine found in nature?
   B.  How does it affect the nervous system_____?

2. Access *www.nida.nih.gov/Alzheimers/publications/medication.html*. Find out the latest drugs approved for the treatment of Alzheimer's disease.

## CRITICAL THINKING

1. It is said that geniuses use approximately 10% of their brain capacity.
   A. About what percentage does the average person use?
   B. What activities can one do to create neuronal connections in the brain?
   C. What is the meaning of the saying, "If you don't use it, you will lose it"?

2. Many people experience a "rush of adrenaline" or a "natural high" from participating in dangerous sports. What does this mean, and what part of the nervous system is affected?

3. You are suddenly called upon in class to make a short oral presentation. Describe what mental and emotional changes are taking place in your mind and body as you prepare to carry out your assignment.

4. How is the blood-brain barrier like a fence around your home?

Copyright © 2007 Elsevier, Inc. All rights reserved.

# 18 Respiratory System

**TERMS AND DEFINITIONS**

Select the correct term from the following list and write the corresponding letter in the blank next to the statement.

A. Asthma

B. COPD

C. Cough reflex

D. Cystic fibrosis

E. Decongestant

F. Expectorant

G. Influenza

H. MDI

I. Nonproductive cough

J. Productive cough

K. Prophylaxis

L. Sputum

M. Viscosity

N. Antitussives

_____ 1. Fluid coughed up from the lungs and bronchial tissues

_____ 2. The thickness of a solution or fluid (e.g., corn syrup is very viscous)

_____ 3. Response of the body intended to clear air passages of foreign substances and mucus by forceful expiration

_____ 4. An inherited disorder that causes production of very thick mucus in the respiratory tract and that affects the pancreas and sweat glands

_____ 5. Medication that prevents or relieves coughing

_____ 6. Metered dose inhaler; a method of supplying medication to the lungs through inhalation

_____ 7. A respiratory tract infection caused by an influenza virus

_____ 8. Drugs that reduce swelling of the mucous membranes by constricting dilated blood vessels, diminishing blood flow to nasal tissues and thereby reducing nasal congestion

_____ 9. Cough that expectorates mucous secretions from the respiratory tract

_____ 10. Chronic obstructive pulmonary disease; a disease process in which the lungs have a decreased capacity for gas exchange; also known as *emphysema* and *chronic bronchitis*

_____ 11. Preventive treatment

_____ 12. Chemical that aids the removal of mucous secretions from the respiratory system by loosening and thinning sputum and bronchial secretions

_____ 13. A condition in which narrowing of the airways impedes breathing

_____ 14. Cough that does not produce mucous secretions (dry cough)

Copyright © 2007 Elsevier, Inc. All rights reserved.

## TRUE OR FALSE

Write T or F next to each statement.

_____ 1. The respiratory rate of a child and an adult are the same.

_____ 2. Both men and women have cartilage around the larynx.

_____ 3. The left bronchus is bigger than the right bronchus.

_____ 4. The diaphragm separates the chest cavity from the abdominal area.

_____ 5. Breathing is an involuntary mechanism.

_____ 6. Viral pneumonia is preventable if a prophylactic vaccine is used.

_____ 7. Smokers may be among those who most often develop bronchitis.

_____ 8. Asthma is classified as an inflammatory lung disease.

_____ 9. Tuberculosis is the most common bacterial disease affecting the pulmonary system.

_____ 10. Individuals who have high blood pressure should take Sudafed regularly.

## SYSTEM IDENTIFIER

Identify each organ in this system and enter the term next to the corresponding number.

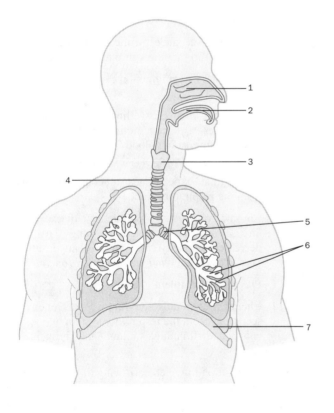

1. _____

2. _____

3. _____

4. _____

5. _____

6. _____

7. _____

## MULTIPLE CHOICE

Complete each question by circling the best answer.

1. The body's pH level must remain close to
   A. 1.7
   B. 5.6
   C. 6.5
   D. 7.4

2. Where does the exchange of gases take place?
   A. Trachea
   B. Bronchi
   C. Bronchioles
   D. Alveolar sacs

**72**

Copyright © 2007 Elsevier, Inc. All rights reserved.

3. Which of the following is *not* a part of the upper respiratory system?
   A. Trachea
   B. Larynx
   C. Pharynx
   D. Nose

4. The windpipe is called the
   A. Trachea
   B. Larynx
   C. Pharynx
   D. Nose

5. The voice box is called the
   A. Trachea
   B. Larynx
   C. Pharynx
   D. Nose

6. Which of the following is *not* a part of the lower respiratory tract?
   A. Larynx
   B. Trachea
   C. Bronchioles
   D. Lungs

7. To relieve a dry, nonproductive cough and to loosen mucus so that it can be expelled through coughing, a patient can take a (an)
   A. Antitussive
   B. Expectorant
   C. Antihistamine
   D. Decongestant

8. Dyspnea is a condition characterized by
   A. Respiration stops
   B. Rapid breathing
   C. Labored or difficult breathing
   D. Lack of breathing that causes the skin to turn blue-gray

9. *Rhinorrhea* is the medical name for a (an)
   A. Allergy
   B. Cold
   C. Sore throat
   D. Runny nose

10. Emphysema can be caused by
    A. Repeated bronchial infections
    B. Smoking
    C. Genetic disposition
    D. All of the above

## FILL IN THE BLANK

1. The act of respiration is broken down into the two distinct phases of _____ and _____.

2. During inspiration, the diaphragm _____, the intercostals _____, and the size of the thoracic cavity _____.

3. The functions of mucous membranes are to _____ and _____ inhaled air.

4. The function of bronchioles is to provide _____ distribution and a passageway for _____ to reach the alveoli.

5. The main function of the lungs is breathing, also known as _____ _____.

6. The respiratory control center is located in the _____ of the brain.

7. The three mechanisms that cause a person to sneeze are _____ _____, _____, and _____.

8. Two common treatments for a cold are _____ and _____.

9. The vaccine that gives immunity for 14 common bacterial pneumonia infections is _____.

10. Three treatments for bronchitis, emphysema, and asthma are _____, _____ and _____.

Copyright © 2007 Elsevier, Inc. All rights reserved.

## MATCHING

### Matching I

Matching the following classes of drugs with their mechanisms of action.

_____ 1. Antitussives

A. Help clear respiratory passages

_____ 2. Mucolytics

B. Act as antiinflammatory agents

_____ 3. Decongestants

C. Break up mucus in patients with COPD and CF

_____ 4. Corticosteroids

D. Inhibit the action of ACh

_____ 5. Anticholinergics

E. Suppress coughing

### Matching II

Match the disease states with their drug treatments.

_____ 1. TB

A. Pseudoephedrine

_____ 2. Chronic asthma

B. Guaifenesin

_____ 3. Cold

C. Isoniazid, rifampin

_____ 4. COPD

D. Azmacort

_____ 5. Cough

E. Acetylcysteine

## RESEARCH ACTIVITY

1. Visit the website _http://www.lungusa.org_. Type the words "secondhand smoke" in the search bar. Read about secondhand smoke and its effects on children.

2. Access the website _www.cdc.gov_. Read the information found under Avian flu virus—Key facts.

3. Access the website _http://www.nlm.nih.gov/medlineplus/cysticfibrosis.html_. Read the information about cystic fibrosis. Whom does this disease affect? What are some of the physical difficulties patients with cystic fibrosis encounter?

## CRITICAL THINKING

1. Smoking has increased dramatically among teenagers over the years. What do you think has been a contributing factor to the increase?

2. What are the health benefits of having plants in your home and office?

3. While having dinner in a restaurant, you see a person who may be choking. You quickly go over to help. What is the first question you should ask the person? Why?

4. Pseudoephedrine now must be sold by a pharmacist, and customers must fill out a log book for their purchase. Why is the sale of pseudoephedrine now controlled?

5. Why do some people become ill with the flu even if they have received the flu vaccine?

Copyright © 2007 Elsevier, Inc. All rights reserved.

# 19 Visual and Auditory Systems

## TERMS AND DEFINITIONS

Select the correct term from the following list and write the corresponding letter in the blank next to the statement.

A. Accommodation

B. Acoustic nerve

C. Aqueous humor

D. Auditory canal

E. Auditory ossicles

F. Cataract

G. Cones

H. Cornea

I. Cycloplegia

J. Eustachian tube

K. Labyrinth

L. Miosis

M. Mydriasis

N. Myopia

O. Ophthalmic

P. Otic

Q. Rods

R. Tympanic membrane

_____ 1. The transparent tissue covering the anterior portion of the eye

_____ 2. Pertaining to the ear

_____ 3. A bony maze composed of the vestibule, cochlea, and semicircular canals of the inner ear

_____ 4. Dilation of the pupil

_____ 5. Pertaining to the eye

_____ 6. Photoreceptors responsible for color (daylight vision)

_____ 7. Paralysis of the ciliary muscle in the eye

_____ 8. A 1-inch segment of tube that runs from the external ear to the middle ear

_____ 9. A membranous skin that separates the external ear from the middle ear

_____ 10. Nearsightedness

_____ 11. Contraction of the pupil

_____ 12. Photoreceptors responsible for black and white colors (night vision) that respond to dim light

_____ 13. The set of three small, bony structures in the ear (i.e., the malleus, incus, and stapes)

_____ 14. The fluid found in the anterior and posterior chambers of the eye

_____ 15. The change that occurs in the ocular lens when it focuses at various distances

_____ 16. Loss of transparency of the lens of the eye

_____ 17. A tubular structure in the middle ear that runs to the nasopharynx (throat)

_____ 18. The cranial nerve that controls the senses of hearing and equilibrium and that eventually leads to the cerebellum and the medulla

Copyright © 2007 Elsevier, Inc. All rights reserved.

## TRUE OR FALSE

Write T or F next to each statement.

_____ 1. The cornea contains blood vessels that provide nourishment to the eye.

_____ 2. The iris is responsible for the color of the eye.

_____ 3. Glaucoma can cause blindness.

_____ 4. About 90% of individuals with glaucoma have open-angle glaucoma.

_____ 5. Color blindness can be treated with surgery.

_____ 6. Ophthalmic erythromycin comes in many dosage forms.

_____ 7. The eustachian tube is located in the middle ear.

_____ 8. Otic agents can increase hearing over time.

_____ 9. An ophthalmic medication commonly is prescribed to treat an otic condition.

_____ 10. Most otic infections require treatment with antiviral agents.

## MULTIPLE CHOICE

Complete each question by circling the best answer.

1. Alteration of which two senses can change a life the most dramatically?
   A. Sight and touch
   B. Smell and taste
   C. Hearing and sight
   D. Smell and hearing

2. A person who is trained to perform an eye examination is called an
   A. Optician
   B. Optometrist
   C. Optimist
   D. Ophthalmologist

3. The purpose of the eyebrow is to
   A. Make the eye more attractive
   B. Trap sweat
   C. Help keep the eyes moist
   D. Shade the eyes from light

4. The lateral rectus rotates
   A. Outward
   B. Inward
   C. Upward and outward
   D. Downward and inward

5. Glaucoma is caused by
   A. Viral infections
   B. Bacterial infections
   C. Increased pressure within the eye
   D. Allergies

6. Which of the following is not a cause of conjunctivitis?
   A. Viral infections
   B. Bacterial infections
   C. Increased pressure within the eye
   D. Allergies

7. Which drug would be indicated for glaucoma?
   A. Propine
   B. Timoptic
   C. Genoptic
   D. Viroptic

8. A possible side effect of Xalatan is
   A. Drowsiness
   B. Nausea and vomiting
   C. Diarrhea
   D. Changes in eye color

9. The eardrum has two major functions; they are
   A. To produce cerumen
   B. To protect the middle ear from foreign objects
   C. To transmit sound toward the middle ear
   D. B and C

10. A ringing or buzzing in the ear is called
    A. Tinnitus
    B. Tendonitis
    C. Rhinitis
    D. Conjunctivitis

11. The part of the eye that contains the enzyme lysozyme and that has antimicrobial properties is the
    A. Retina
    B. Sclera
    C. Lacrimal gland (tears)
    D. Conjunctiva

12. The _____ contain(s) the receptors for vision.
    A. Choroids
    B. Cornea
    C. Vitreous body
    D. Retina

Copyright © 2007 Elsevier, Inc. All rights reserved.

## FILL IN THE BLANK

1. An alternative to wearing glasses is _____ surgery.

2. Two new treatments to reverse the effects of blindness are _____ and _____.

3. Three common ophthalmic dosage forms are _____, _____, and _____.

4. CAIs are used as a long-term treatment for _____ _____ _____, whereas mitotics are used only preoperatively for individuals with _____ _____ _____.

5. Most of the agents used to reduce inflammation are _____ and _____ (dosage forms).

6. Decongestants and antihistamines are used to combat _____.

7. Three common viral infections of the eye are _____, _____, and _____.

8. The three main functions of the ear are _____, _____, and _____.

9. The fluid-filled inner ear is called the _____; it transmits sound via _____ _____ to the brain.

10. Deafness caused by factors other than genetic abnormalities includes _____ and _____.

11. Pediatricians insert _____ _____ in the ears of children who suffer from chronic _____ _____.

12. Almost all ear agents contain a combination of _____ and _____ agents to remove wax buildup.

## MATCHING

### Matching I
Match the following trade and generic drug names.

_____ 1. Trusopt     A. Latanoprost

_____ 2. Xalatan     B. Dexamethasone

_____ 3. Voltaren     C. Tobramycin

_____ 4. Decadron     D. Dorzolamide

_____ 5. TobraDex     E. Diclofenac

### Matching II
Match the following medications with the ear conditions they treat.

1. _____ Glycerin     A. External ear infections

2. _____ Desonide     B. Pain associated with swimmer's ear

3. _____ Acetic acid     C. Bacterial ear infections

4. _____ Polymyxin     D. Ear wax

5. _____ Benzocaine     E. Swimmer's ear

## RESEARCH ACTIVITY

1. Visit a local pharmacy and locate the eye and ear sections.
   A. What is the main ingredient in OTC eye drops?
   B. What is the main ingredient in OTC ear drops?

Copyright © 2007 Elsevier, Inc. All rights reserved.

2. Access the website *http://www.lighthouse.org/sharing_solutions_spring2001_eye_disease_treatment. htm*. What are the latest developments in the treatment of eye disease?

## CRITICAL THINKING

1. You been working in the IV room all day, and your eyes are feeling very dry. What is the reason for your "dry eyes," and what can you do to resolve the situation?

2. Night blindness is often caused by a lack of vitamin A. What food can you eat to prevent night blindness?

3. Your child came home from school with pinkeye. How can you prevent yourself from getting this contagious eye infection?

4. Why is NaCl an ingredient in every artificial tear product?

5. How is having an inner ear infection different from having a middle ear infection?

Copyright © 2007 Elsevier, Inc. All rights reserved.

# 20 Gastrointestinal System

## TERMS AND DEFINITIONS

Select the correct term from the following list and write the corresponding letter in the blank next to the statement.

A. Absorption

B. Amino acids

C. Appendicitis

D. Carbohydrates

E. Chyme

F. Constipation

G. Diarrhea

H. Digestion

I. Emesis

J. Excretion

K. Gastritis

L. Peptic ulcer

M. Ingestion

N. Lipids

O. Peristalsis

P. Ulcer

Q. Villus

_____ 1. Inflammation of the appendix

_____ 2. Fats and fatty acids

_____ 3. Frequent, watery, loose stools

_____ 4. Inflammation of the stomach lining

_____ 5. A lesion on a mucous surface of the gastrointestinal (GI) tract

_____ 6. Molecules that make up proteins

_____ 7. An ulcerative condition of the lower esophagus, stomach, or duodenum usually caused by the bacterium *Helicobacter pylori (H. pylori)*

_____ 8. Vomiting

_____ 9. The taking in of nutrients from food and liquids

_____ 10. The soupy consistency of food after it has mixed with stomach acids and as it passes into the small intestine

_____ 11. Chemical substances made up of only carbon, hydrogen, and oxygen (e.g., sugars, starches, and cellulose)

_____ 12. To take in food or liquid

_____ 13. A projection from the surface of a mucous membrane

_____ 14. Elimination of waste products through stools and urine

_____ 15. The mechanical, chemical, and enzymatic action of breaking down food into molecules that can be used in metabolism

_____ 16. The contraction and relaxation of the tubular molecules of the esophagus, stomach, and intestines that move food from the mouth to the anus

_____ 17. The presence of dry, hard stools that may be decreased in frequency

Copyright © 2007 Elsevier, Inc. All rights reserved.

## TRUE OR FALSE

Write T or F next to each statement.

_____ 1. All medications used to treat symptoms of the digestive tract and intestines are prescription only.

_____ 2. The GI system is controlled by the sympathetic system.

_____ 3. The pharynx connects the mouth to the esophagus.

_____ 4. The small intestine is about 6 feet in length.

_____ 5. The small intestine is connected to the liver and the pancreas.

_____ 6. The gallbladder aids digestion by releasing bile.

_____ 7. The colon is the shortest section of the intestinal tract.

_____ 8. The appendix plays a vital role in the digestive system.

_____ 9. The mouth comes in contact with many kinds of bacteria every day.

_____ 10. Proton pump inhibitors, such as $H_2$-antagonists, are available in lesser strengths over the counter.

## SYSTEM IDENTIFIER

Identify each organ in this system and enter the term next to the corresponding number.

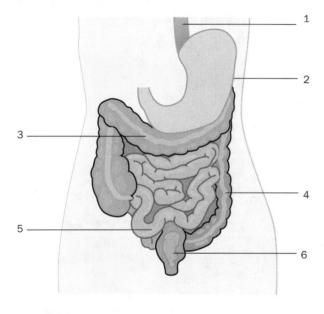

1. _____
2. _____
3. _____
4. _____
5. _____
6. _____

## MULTIPLE CHOICE

Complete each question by circling the best answer.

1. Which of the following is *not* a main function of the GI system?
   A. Digestion
   B. Absorption
   C. Metabolism
   D. Production of flatus

2. Which of the following is *not* a salivary gland?
   A. Subcutaneous
   B. Sublingual
   C. Submandibular
   D. Parotid

3. The function of the epiglottis is to close off the _____ so that food does not enter the wrong tube.
   A. Pharynx
   B. Trachea
   C. Esophagus
   D. Colon

4. Most absorption takes place in the
   A. Duodenum
   B. Jejunum
   C. Ileum
   D. All of the above

Copyright © 2007 Elsevier, Inc. All rights reserved.

5. The main sections of the large intestines are the
   A. Cecum and ileum
   B. Rectum and jejunum
   C. Colon and rectum
   D. A and B

6. Which of the following is *not* a common condition that affects the GI system?
   A. Heartburn
   B. Appendicitis
   C. Constipation
   D. Diarrhea

7. The abbreviated term *s/s* means
   A. Swish and swallow
   B. Sit and spin
   C. Swish and spit
   D. A and C

8. Simethicone is indicated for
   A. Flatulence
   B. Diarrhea
   C. Heartburn
   D. Constipation

9. Aluminum can cause
   A. Flatulence
   B. Diarrhea
   C. Heartburn
   D. Constipation

10. A patient has vomiting; the physician may prescribe
    A. Axid
    B. Colace
    C. Compazine
    D. Lomotil

## FILL IN THE BLANK

1. The act of building molecules is known as _____, and the act of breaking down molecules to release energy is called _____.

2. The environment of the stomach is a more _____ pH, and the environment of the intestines is a more _____ pH.

3. Lack of good _____ hygiene is the most common reason conditions affecting the mouth occur.

4. Symptoms of inflammation include _____ and _____.

5. Treatments for the mouth include _____, _____, _____, and _____.

6. Two conditions caused by hyperacidity are _____ and _____ ulcers.

7. GERD and heartburn can be treated with _____ and _____.

8. The most effective combination of medications for *H. pylori* is _____, _____, _____, and _____.

9. One of the most common causes of diarrhea and constipation is _____.

10. Kaopectate, Fibercon, and PeptoBismol, used to treat diarrhea, are available _____.

11. An example of a gentle laxative is _____ powder, and an example of a harsh laxative is _____.

12. A common side effect of chemotherapy is _____.

## MATCHING

**Matching I**
Match the following trade and generic drug names.

_____ 1. Pepcid          A. Bisacodyl

_____ 2. Prevacid        B. Loperamide

_____ 3. Dulcolax        C. Famotidine

_____ 4. Imodium         D. Prochlorperazine

_____ 5. Compazine       E. Lansoprazole

**Matching II**
Match the following drug classes with the correct example.

_____ 1. Tagamet         A. Antidiarrheal

_____ 2. Prilosec        B. Antiemetic

_____ 3. Fibercon        C. H$_2$-antagonist

_____ 4. Reglan          D. Emetic

_____ 5. Ipecac          E. Proton pump inhibitor

Copyright © 2007 Elsevier, Inc. All rights reserved.

## SHORT ANSWER

1. What is the sequence of organs in the gastrointestinal tract? _____
_____

2. What is the important function of the instrinsic factor found in the stomach? _____
_____

## RESEARCH ACTIVITY

1. Many prescription medications for GI upset and heartburn have been changed to OTC status. Visit the website *www.fda.gov* and make a list of (a) the GI medications that are now available OTC and (b) the difference in dosage strengths compared with when these drugs were prescription medications.

2. Visit the website *www.cvs.com*. Compare the prices of the medications you listed in question 1.

## CRITICAL THINKING

1. It has been stated that you must chew your food "32 times." How does not chewing your food affect digestion in the stomach?

2. A hectic and stressful lifestyle can produce many "stomach problems," such as indigestion, gastritis, and peptic ulcers. What lifestyle changes can you make to prevent these problems?

3. What constitutes good oral hygiene? Is flossing that important?

4. Many articles recommend drinking eight glasses of water a day. What are some of the benefits of doing so?

5. Is bulimia a psychological or a physical condition?

Copyright © 2007 Elsevier, Inc. All rights reserved.

# 21 Urinary System

## TERMS AND DEFINITIONS

Select the correct term from the following list and write the corresponding letter in the blank next to the statement.

A. Acidification

B. Acidosis

C. Alkalosis

D. Blood urea nitrogen (BUN)

E. Congestive heart failure (CHF)

F. Diuresis

G. Diuretics

H. Edema

I. Excretion

J. Hyperkalemia

K. Hypokalemia

L. Incontinence

M. Micturition

N. Nocturia

O. Pyelonephritis

P. Urinary retention

Q. Urea

R. Uremia

S. Urolithiasis

T. Dialysis

_____ 1. Inability to empty the bladder completely

_____ 2. A local or generalized condition in which body tissues retain an excessive amount of fluid

_____ 3. A test that measures nitrogen in the blood in the form of urea

_____ 4. Loss of control over excretion of urine or feces

_____ 5. An agent that increases urine output and diuresis

_____ 6. Inflammation of the kidney and renal pelvis

_____ 7. Kidney stones

_____ 8. An abnormally low concentration of potassium in the blood

_____ 9. Accumulation of blood in the circulatory system caused by insufficient pumping of the heart

_____ 10. Conversion to an acid environment

_____ 11. Secretion and passage of large amounts of urine from the body

_____ 12. Urination

_____ 13. An increase in the alkalinity of the blood caused by the accumulation of alkalies or a reduction of acid content; the result is a rise in the pH of the blood

_____ 14. The main nitrogenous constituent of urine and final product of protein metabolism; it is formed in the liver

_____ 15. Elimination of waste products from the body

_____ 16. The buildup in the body of urea and other nitrogenous compounds that normally would be excreted by healthy kidneys

_____ 17. Passage of a solute through a semipermeable membrane to remove toxic materials and to maintain fluids, electrolytes, and the pH of the body system when the kidneys no longer work

_____ 18. The need to urinate excessively at night

_____ 19. An increase in the acid content of the blood caused by the accumulation of acid or a loss of bicarbonate; as a result, the pH of the blood is lowered

_____ 20. An excessive amount of potassium in the blood

Copyright © 2007 Elsevier, Inc. All rights reserved.

## TRUE OR FALSE

Write T or F next to each statement.

_____ 1. The shape of the kidneys is similar to the shape of a kidney bean.

_____ 2. When the kidney is full, the person feels the urge to urinate.

_____ 3. The body excretes about 960 mL of urine per day.

_____ 4. Hemoglobin gives blood its red color.

_____ 5. The ureter tubes lead to the bladder.

_____ 6. It is impossible for people to survive without two functioning kidneys.

_____ 7. Drinking plenty of water is one of the most effective ways to take care of the urinary system.

_____ 8. Younger adults suffer from acute renal failure more often than older people.

_____ 9. Men are more susceptible to UTIs than are women.

_____ 10. Incontinence tends to affect women more than men.

## SYSTEM IDENTIFIER

Identify each component in this system and enter the term next to the corresponding number.

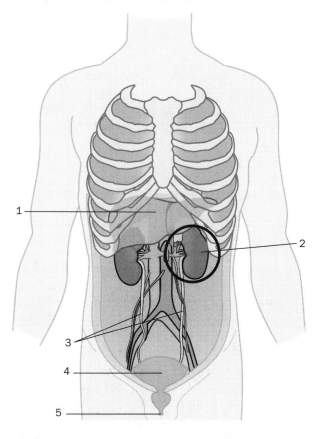

1. _____

2. _____

3. _____

4. _____

5. _____

## MULTIPLE CHOICE

Complete each question by circling the best answer.

1. The urge to urinate is called
   A. Maturation
   B. Micturition
   C. Acidification
   D. Excretion

2. What volume of blood products do the kidneys filter each day?
   A. 0.5 gallons
   B. 5 gallons
   C. 50 gallons
   D. 500 gallons

Copyright © 2007 Elsevier, Inc. All rights reserved.

3. Albumins and globulins are components of
   A. Plasma
   B. Blood
   C. Hemoglobin
   D. All of the above

4. The one-way reabsorption of sodium and chloride from the loop of Henle is called
   A. Ion exchange
   B. Osmosis
   C. Active transport
   D. Tubular secretion

5. The productions of a large volume of urine within a certain period of time is called
   A. Anuria
   B. Oliguria
   C. Polyuria
   D. Uremia

6. Which of the following is a symptom of end-stage renal disease?
   A. CHF
   B. Pulmonary edema
   C. Nausea and vomiting
   D. All of the above

7. A nosocomial infection is an infection
   A. Of the nose
   B. Acquired in the hospital
   C. Acquired while in a coma
   D. None of the above

8. Which of the following is *not* a means of cleansing the blood of patients with ESRD?
   A. Hemodialysis
   B. Peritoneal dialysis
   C. Nocturnal dialysis
   D. Oxydialysis

9. The most common side effect of all thiazide-like agents is
   A. Frequent urination
   B. Infrequent urination
   C. Increased thiamine levels
   D. Decreased thiamine levels

10. Kegel exercises are done to help overcome
    A. Stress
    B. Incontinence
    C. CHF
    D. UTIs

## FILL IN THE BLANK

1. The four major functions of the body are _____, _____, _____, and _____.

2. _____ occurs when too many free hydrogen ions are present, and _____ occurs when too many hydroxide ions are present.

3. The portion of the kidneys that actually does the work of separation is the _____.

4. Two important functions of the nephron are _____ and _____.

5. The acid content in urine is between pH _____.

6. An example of a buffer is _____.

7. Two causes of edema are _____ and _____.

8. One of the most common conditions affecting the urinary system is _____.

9. People receiving dialysis must watch their _____ and _____.

10. The mechanism of action for thiazides and thiazide-like agents is that they equally _____ the urinary excretion of the ions _____ and _____.

## SHORT ANSWER

1. Name the six main types of drugs used to treat edema.

_____    _____    _____

_____    _____    _____

2. What are the symptoms of an upper UTI and a lower UTI?

Upper: _____

Lower: _____

3. Who is at high risk for renal failure? _____, _____, _____, _____, and _____

Copyright © 2007 Elsevier, Inc. All rights reserved.

## MATCHING

### Matching I

Match the following medical terms with their definitions.

_____ 1. Anuria     A. Inflammation of the urethra

_____ 2. Cystitis     B. Inflammation of the kidney

_____ 3. Urethritis     C. Excessive decrease in potassium in the blood

_____ 4. Hypokalemia     D. Lack of urine

_____ 5. Pyelonephritis     E. Inflammation of the bladder

### Matching II

Match the following trade names with their generic drug names.

_____ 1. Diuril     A. Spironolactone

_____ 2. Lasix     B. Acetazolamide

_____ 3. Aldactone     C. Chlorothiazide

_____ 4. Diamox     D. Nitrofurantoin

_____ 5. Macrodantin     E. Furosemide

## RESEARCH ACTIVITY

1. Visit the website *http://www.healthandage.com/PHome/gm=2!gid2=1332*. Investigate the benefits of cranberries for the treatment of urinary tract infections.

2. At the website *http://www.yoga-for-health-and-fitness.com/benefits-of-drinking-water.htm*, investigate the benefits of drinking eight glasses of water a day.

3. Access the website *http://seniors-site.com/ultimate/dialysis.html*. Read the information about dialysis treatment.

## CRITICAL THINKING

1. Methicillin-resistant *Staphylococcus aureus* (MRSA) is a well-known nosocomial infection. Patients in the intensive care unit are quite susceptible to MRSA. What are some ways to prevent the spread of this type of infection?

2. If a urinary tract infection is left untreated, how will the infection progress?

3. Diabetes can be complicated by hypertension and kidney failure. A change in the patient's diet is always recommended. Apply your knowledge of the disease and devise a list of lifestyle changes that would benefit a diabetic patient.

Copyright © 2007 Elsevier, Inc. All rights reserved.

# 22 Cardiovascular System

●

## TERMS AND DEFINITIONS

Select the correct term from the following list and write the corresponding letter in the blank next to the statement.

A. Arrhythmia

B. Artery

C. Capillary

D. Coagulate

E. Diuretics

F. Edema

G. Enzymes

H. Thrombin

I. Thrombolytic

J. Vein

_____ 1. Medication used to break up a thrombus or blood clot

_____ 2. A vessel that carries oxygenated blood from the heart to the tissues of the body

_____ 3. A condition in which the body tissues contain an excessive amount of fluid

_____ 4. An agent that increases urine secretion

_____ 5. A vessel that carries deoxygenated blood to the heart

_____ 6. To solidify, or to change from a fluid state to a solid state

_____ 7. Proteins that act as a catalyst, causing metabolic reactions to take place at a faster rate in the body

_____ 8. Loss of rhythm; irregular heartbeats

_____ 9. An enzyme formed in coagulating blood that forms blood clots

_____ 10. An extremely small vessel that connects the ends of the smallest arteries to the smallest veins, where the exchange of nutrients and waste, oxygen, and carbon dioxide occurs

## TRUE OR FALSE

Write T or F next to each statement.

_____ 1. A normal heart beats 160 to 200 times per minute.

_____ 2. The right atrium receives oxygenated blood from the lungs and pumps it out to the body.

_____ 3. The cardiac conduction system provides the electrical charge that makes the heart pump.

_____ 4. Most of the body's blood supply is cycled through the heart in 1 minute.

_____ 5. Congestive heart failure is a condition in which the heart cannot pump as vigorously as necessary to deliver blood throughout the body.

_____ 6. The good cholesterol is known as *LDL*.

_____ 7. High blood pressure is also known as the "silent killer" because it has no obvious signs.

_____ 8. Nitroglycerin is good for only 6 months after the container is opened.

_____ 9. Hypotension is more common than hypertension.

_____ 10. Diet and exercise can lower lipid content.

Copyright © 2007 Elsevier, Inc. All rights reserved.

Identify each component in this system and enter the term next to the corresponding number.

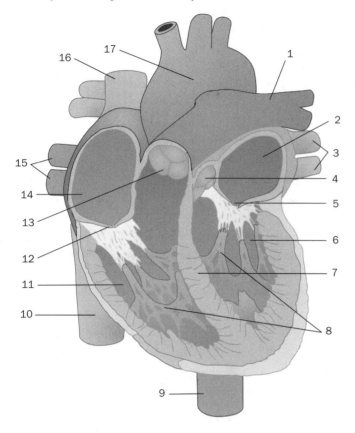

1. _____

2. _____

3. _____

4. _____

5. _____

6. _____

7. _____

8. _____

9. _____

10. _____

11. _____

12. _____

13. _____

14. _____

15. _____

16. _____

17. _____

## MULTIPLE CHOICE

Complete each question by circling the best answer.

1. Tenormin, Inderal, and Lopressor are all classified as
   A. ACE inhibitors
   B. Beta blockers
   C. Calcium channel blockers
   D. Antianginals

2. Which of the following is *not* a main layer of the heart?
   A. Endocardium
   B. Myocardium
   C. Subcardium
   D. Epicardium

3. Pain and pressure in the chest caused by a lack of blood flow and oxygenation of the heart muscle are features of
   A. Angina pectoris
   B. Arrhythmia
   C. Hyperlipidemia
   D. Myocardial infarction

4. Which of the following is *not* a greater risk factor for hypertension?
   A. Age
   B. Gender
   C. Race
   D. None of the above

5. An *embolus* is a
   A. Blood clot
   B. Hemorrhage
   C. Rise in blood pressure
   D. Rise in lipid levels

6. Lovastatin, simvastatin, and pravastatin are classified as
   A. Antihypertensives
   B. Antiarrhythmics
   C. Anticoagulants
   D. Antihyperlipidemics

Copyright © 2007 Elsevier, Inc. All rights reserved.

7. A code blue situation occurs when a patient
   A. Is having a heart attack
   B. Quits breathing
   C. A and B
   D. None of the above

8. An antidote for an overdose of Lanoxin is
   A. Digoxin
   B. Digibind
   C. Digitalis
   D. Digitonin

9. Which of the following is *not* an element of the four-step approach to controlling HBP?
   A. Weight reduction
   B. Diuretics

C. Antianginals
D. Beta blockers

10. Nitrostat tablets should be administered by which route?
    A. PO
    B. SL
    C. SQ
    D. PR

## FILL IN THE BLANK

1. The main arteries that supply blood to the heart are called _____
   _____.

2. Coronary artery disease is associated with _____.

3. A thrombus can cause a _____.

4. Cholesterol is important for the making of _____ and
   _____.

5. A cholesterol level below _____ indicates overall low cholesterol.

6. Two drugs available OTC that can affect BP are _____ and _____.

7. Nitrates are used in the treatment of _____.

8. A _____ is caused by an _____ blood vessel in the brain.

9. _____ and _____ are two side effects of hypotension.

10. Niacin available OTC can lower _____.

## MATCHING

Match the classes of drugs.

_____ 1. Antihyperlipidemics          A. Quinidine, procainamide, verapamil

_____ 2. Arrhythmic agents            B. Heparin, warfarin

_____ 3. Cardioglycosides             C. ACE inhibitors, beta blockers, calcium channel blockers

_____ 4. Antihypertensives            D. Bile acid sequestrants, HMG-CoA reductase inhibitors

_____ 5. Anticoagulants               E. Digoxin

## DRUG NAMES

Give the generic names for the following drugs.

1. Mevacor _____       6. Hytrin _____

2. Norpace _____       7. Quinidex _____

3. Lanoxin _____       8. Zestril _____

4. Dyrenium _____       9. Cozaar _____

5. Lotensin _____      10. Cardizem _____

Copyright © 2007 Elsevier, Inc. All rights reserved.

## EXPLAIN

1. How do ACE inhibitors help reduce BP?

_____

_____

2. How do calcium channel blockers work?

_____

_____

## RESEARCH ACTIVITY

1. Access the website *www.americanheart.org*. What is *tPA*? How does this drug help stroke victims recover?

2. Access the website *www.rxlist.com*. Locate Side Effects and Drug Interactions. What are the side effects of aspirin, and with what drugs does it interact?

## CRITICAL THINKING

1. "An aspirin a day keeps a heart attack away." What are some everyday activities people can do to "keep a heart attack away"?

2. You have just finished your lunch, which consisted of a double cheeseburger, extra large fries, and a cola. Name all the body systems that will be affected by that "yummy" meal.

3. When people are asked to change their lifestyle as a result of life-threatening diseases (such as after an MI), what two words do they dread hearing?

4. "I feel like I'm having a heart attack," someone says to you. How do you know for sure? For what symptoms do you look?

**90**

Chapter **22** **Cardiovascular System**

Copyright © 2007 Elsevier, Inc. All rights reserved.

# 23 Reproductive System

## TERMS AND DEFINITIONS

Select the correct term from the following list and write the corresponding letter in the blank next to the statement.

A. Endometriosis

B. Endometrium

C. Fallopian tubes

D. Fertilization

E. Gametes

F. Inert ingredient

G. Menopause

H. Negative feedback

I. Oocyte or ova

J. Palliative

K. Therapeutic

L. Abortifacients

M. Amenorrhea

N. Androgens

O. Benign prostatic hypertrophy

P. Chloasma

Q. Depot

R. Dysmenorrhea

_____ 1. Brings relief but does not cure

_____ 2. Mucous membrane lining of the uterus

_____ 3. The female reproductive germ cell

_____ 4. An ingredient that has little or no effect on body functions

_____ 5. The narrow passage between the ovary and the uterus

_____ 6. Curative treatment

_____ 7. Sex cells, or ova and sperm

_____ 8. The process by which a sperm unites with an ovum to create a new life

_____ 9. A self-regulating mechanism in which the output of a system has input or control over the process

_____ 10. A condition in which tissue resembling endometrium is found outside the uterine cavity, usually in the pelvic area

_____ 11. Cessation of menstruation; a natural phenomenon in which a woman passes from a reproductive state to a nonreproductive state

_____ 12. Painful menstruation

_____ 13. Any treatment that causes abortion of a fetus

_____ 14. Male hormones

_____ 15. An area of the body where a substance can accumulate or be stored for later distribution

_____ 16. Absence or suppression of menses

_____ 17. Hyperpigmentation of skin, limited or confined to a certain area, that usually is found on the face during pregnancy

_____ 18. Nonmalignant enlargement of the prostate gland

Copyright © 2007 Elsevier, Inc. All rights reserved.

## TRUE OR FALSE

Write T or F next to each statement.

_____ 1. The reproductive system is not interdependent on other body systems.

_____ 2. The gonads provide characteristics of both males and females.

_____ 3. The male reproductive system is closely tied to the endocrine system.

_____ 4. Women produce ova every month.

_____ 5. The female uterus houses the fertilized ovum.

_____ 6. Mammary gland tissue is regulated by hormonal secretions.

_____ 7. The hypothalamus can distinguish between natural and synthetic hormones.

_____ 8. Natural testosterone used for medicinal purposes is obtained from the testes of horses.

_____ 9. Oral contraceptives provide protection from sexually transmitted diseases.

_____ 10. The morning-after pill is a high-dose contraceptive.

## SYSTEM IDENTIFIER

### Male Reproductive System

Identify each component in this system and enter the term next to the corresponding number.

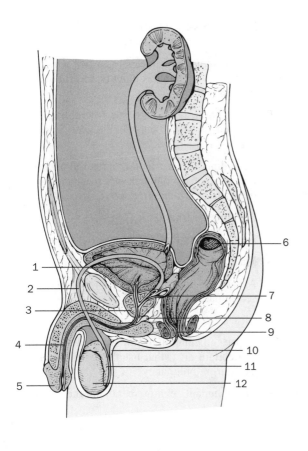

1. _____

2. _____

3. _____

4. _____

5. _____

6. _____

7. _____

8. _____

9. _____

10. _____

11. _____

12. _____

Copyright © 2007 Elsevier, Inc. All rights reserved.

**Female Reproductive System**

Identify each component in this system and enter the term next to the corresponding number.

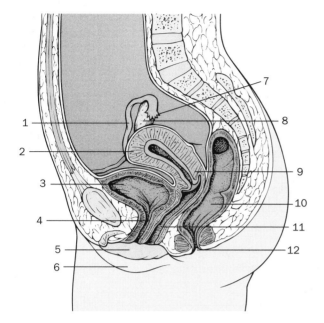

1. _____

2. _____

3. _____

4. _____

5. _____

6. _____

7. _____

8. _____

9. _____

10. _____

11. _____

12. _____

## MULTIPLE CHOICE

Complete each question by circling the best answer.

1. The gonads or reproductive organs are responsible for
   A. Secretion of hormones
   B. Production of sex cells
   C. Gender characteristics of males
   D. A and B

2. Sperm production in males begins at puberty and continues until
   A. Midlife
   B. Age 70
   C. Throughout the lifetime
   D. None of the above

3. The most abundant androgen is
   A. Estrogen
   B. Testosterone
   C. Progesterone
   D. Inhibin

4. The ovum is fertilized in the
   A. Uterus
   B. Cervix
   C. Ovary
   D. Fallopian tube

5. Female hormones are used to treat conditions of the male reproductive tract such as
   A. Prostate cancer
   B. Testicular cancer
   C. Impotence
   D. A and B

6. Oral contraceptives are formulated in which of the following combinations?
   A. Monophasic
   B. Biphasic
   C. Triphasic
   D. All of the above

7. The goal of treatment for benign prostatic hypertrophy is to
   A. Relieve hesitancy of urination
   B. Decrease nocturia
   C. Relieve urinary tract infections
   D. All of the above

8. Which of the following hormones is used to treat abnormal uterine bleeding, abnormal ovulation, and infertility?
   A. Progesterone
   B. Estrogen
   C. Testosterone
   D. Follicle-stimulating hormone

9. The source of estradiol used for hormone replacement therapy is
   A. Plants
   B. Urine of pregnant mares
   C. Placentas
   D. B and C

10. Contraceptives given by injection prevent pregnancy by
    A. Suppressing ovulation
    B. Thickening the cervical mucus
    C. Altering the endometrium
    D. All of the above

Copyright © 2007 Elsevier, Inc. All rights reserved.

Chapter **23**  **Reproductive System**

## FILL IN THE BLANK

1. Patients taking _____ should not take sildenafil because it causes a dangerous decrease in blood pressure.

2. _____ is known as the abortion pill.

3. One cause of infertility is _____.

4. The barrier types of contraceptives for females are _____, _____, and _____.

5. Latex, polyurethane, and lamb intestine are the three types of materials used to make _____.

6. The side effects of _____ _____ include thromboembolism, increased myocardial infarctions, and strokes.

7. The side effects of _____ include weight gain, stomach pain, and stomach cramping.

8. _____ are one of the natural sources from which progestins can be obtained.

9. Oil-based estrogen medications are called _____ medications.

10. Female hormones are in a _____ pattern every month.

## MATCHING

### Matching I
Match the following trade and generic drug names.

____ 1. Proscar      A. Conjugated estrogens

____ 2. Flomax      B. Estropipate

____ 3. Premarin      C. Finasteride

____ 4. Ogen      D. Medroxyprogesterone

____ 5. Provera      E. Tamsulosin

### Matching II
Match the following trade and generic drug names.

____ 1. Parlodel      A. Ethinyl estradiol/ norgestrel

____ 2. Ortho Tri-Cyclen      B. Sildenafil

____ 3. Lo-Ovral      C. Terazosin

____ 4. Hytrin      D. Bromocriptine

____ 5. Viagra      E. Ethinyl estradiol/ norgestimate

## SHORT ANSWER

1. Sildenafil (Viagra) was introduced in 1998 for the treatment of _____. Today it is used for _____ _____.

2. Any disease that can be transmitted by _____ _____ is considered an STD.

3. Clotrimazole is used as a treatment for what fungal infection? _____ _____.

4. Combination oral contraceptives consist of both _____ and _____, which act to inhibit ovulation.

5. The primary actions of estrogens are to maintain reproductive structures such as _____ and to _____.

6. In males, androgens stimulate the formation of _____ _____ _____ like increased _____ and growth of _____ _____.

Copyright © 2007 Elsevier, Inc. All rights reserved.

1. Access the website *www.birthcontrol.com*. Research the latest developments in birth control for both males and females.

2. Access the website *www.niaid.nih.gov/factsheet/stdpid.htm*. Read about pelvic inflammatory disease and its effects on sexually active young women.

3. Access the website *http://webmd.lycos.com*. Type in "saw palmetto." Read the article, "An Herb for Prostate Problems?"

## CRITICAL THINKING

1. Women have been told for many years that when menopause occurs, they will need hormonal replacement therapy. However, recently released information indicates that hormonal replacement therapy is more harmful than beneficial. What advice will you give women on this subject?

2. Birth control has been taught in middle schools and high schools for many years in an attempt to curb teen pregnancy. Why is the rate of teen pregnancy still high?

3. Rogaine was approved by the FDA for the treatment of hair loss in 1998. The active ingredient in Rogaine is finasteride, the same drug that is used to treat benign prostatic hypertrophy. What is the difference in strength between Rogaine and the prescription form of finasteride, and what are the side effects of this drug?

Copyright © 2007 Elsevier, Inc. All rights reserved.

# 24 Antiinfectives

## TERMS AND DEFINITIONS

Select the correct term from the following list and write the corresponding letter in the blank next to the statement.

A. Antibiotic
B. Antimicrobial
C. Bacteria
D. Bactericidal
E. Bacteriostatic
F. Fungicide
G. Gram-negative bacteria
H. Gram-positive bacteria
I. Helminth
J. Inhibit
K. Morphology
L. Mycosis
M. Normal flora
N. Nosocomial infection
O. Parasites
P. Protozoa
Q. PRSP
R. Synthesis
S. Symbiotic
T. Viruses
U. Vector

_____ 1. Unicellular organisms

_____ 2. Organisms that cannot replicate without the necessary components from a host

_____ 3. Bacteria that are unable to keep crystal violet stain when washed in acid alcohol

_____ 4. Kingdom *protista;* unicellular organism

_____ 5. Fungal disease

_____ 6. Appearance of an organism, including its shape, size, structure, and Gram staining characteristics

_____ 7. The formation of chemical components in the body systems that comprise cell contents or containers

_____ 8. Agents that prevent the growth of bacteria but do not kill the microbe

_____ 9. A living entity that can transmit an infective organism but that does not itself have the disease (e.g., the role of the mosquito in the transmission of malaria)

_____ 10. Chemical agents produced by scientists to prevent growth or to kill

_____ 11. Any type of infection a person acquires while hospitalized

_____ 12. Multicellular worms

_____ 13. A close relationship between two species

_____ 14. Agents that kill bacteria

_____ 15. Microorganisms that reside harmlessly in the body and do not cause disease, but rather may aid the host organism

_____ 16. Chemical agents produced by organisms used to treat infection

_____ 17. To stop or hold back in order to prevent a reaction from taking place

_____ 18. Agents that kill fungi

_____ 19. Penicillin-resistant *Streptococcus pneumoniae*

_____ 20. Bacteria that are able to keep crystal violet stain when washed in acid alcohol

_____ 21. Organisms that require a host for nourishment and reproduction

97

Copyright © 2007 Elsevier, Inc. All rights reserved.

## TRUE OR FALSE

Write T or F next to each statement.

_____ 1. The immune system identifies and kills foreign bodies that have invaded the body.

_____ 2. As patients begin to feel better, they should stop taking their antibiotics.

_____ 3. Penicillins have a more effective bactericidal action on gram-negative bacteria.

_____ 4. Microorganisms have the ability to alter their genetic makeup.

_____ 5. Infections can appear anywhere on or in the body.

_____ 6. Nosocomial infections can be deadly.

_____ 7. Fungi grow only on people who live in moist, warm climates.

_____ 8. Viruses are organisms that live outside their host.

_____ 9. HIV is the precursor to AIDS.

_____ 10. Roundworms can be transferred in undercooked meat.

## MULTIPLE CHOICE

Complete each question by circling the best answer.

1. Which of the following is *not* a common type of microorganism?
   A. Bacteria
   B. Fungi
   C. AIDS
   D. Protozoa

2. The main area susceptible to infection is the
   A. Genitals
   B. GI tract
   C. Lungs
   D. All of the above

3. One of the major infections that affects the stomach is
   A. Chlamydia
   B. *H. pylori*
   C. Tinea
   D. Meningitis

4. Which of the following is *not* a common symptom of a respiratory infection?
   A. Wheezing
   B. Coughing
   C. Hiccups
   D. Shortness of breath

5. Tuberculosis affects the
   A. Respiratory system
   B. Cardiovascular system
   C. Urinary tract
   D. Gastrointestinal system

6. Individuals at high risk for skin infections are
   A. Dialysis patients
   B. Diabetic patients
   C. Elderly patients
   D. Pediatric patients

7. Keflex and Suprax are classified as
   A. Penicillins
   B. Aminoglycosides

C. Cephalosporins
D. Antiprotozoans

8. Aminoglycosides can be dangerous because
   A. They come in IV form only
   B. They are given q4h
   C. They are addictive
   D. A narrow range exists between therapeutic and toxic dosages

9. *Candida* infections can occur
   A. In the mouth
   B. In the vagina
   C. Under the nails
   D. All of the above

10. Which of the following is *not* a way that malaria can be transmitted?
    A. Unprotected sex
    B. Infected needles
    C. Mosquitos
    D. Blood

11. What allows a microorganism to decrease the action of antibiotics?
    A. Environment
    B. Resistance
    C. Overuse
    D. None of the above

12. Two compounds added to amoxicillin and ampicillin to strengthen them against microbe resistance are
    A. Hydrochloric acid and sodium chloride
    B. Neosporin and bacitracin
    C. Clavulanate acid and sulbactam
    D. Sodium bicarbonate and Azactam

13. Which of the following organisms is *not* a cause of STDs?
    A. Bacteria
    B. Protozoa
    C. Fungi
    D. Viruses

Copyright © 2007 Elsevier, Inc. All rights reserved.

## FILL IN THE BLANK

1. Three antibiotics used to treat *H. pylori* infection of the stomach are _____, _____ _____, and _____.

2. TB is diagnosed by a tuberculin _____ but must be confirmed by a _____ _____ that isolates the bacterium.

3. The two most common fungal infections are _____ _____ and _____ _____.

4. The most common eye infection is _____.

5. Antibiotics are often referred to as _____ spectrum and _____ spectrum.

6. The mechanism of action of penicillin is bacteriocidal toward microbes that are _____ _____.

7. Two main infections in humans caused by a mycobacterium are _____ and _____.

8. The mechanism of action of parenteral aminoglycosides is their ability to _____ to the ribosomes of microorganisms, stopping _____ synthesis.

9. Tinea pedis is also known as _____ _____.

10. Viruses require a host's DNA to _____.

## SHORT ANSWER

Give examples of drugs from the following drug classes.

1. First-generation penicillin _____

2. Penicillinase resistant _____

3. Cephalosporins: first generation _____, second generation _____ _____, third generation _____, fourth generation _____

4. Aminoglycoside _____

5. Antiprotozoan _____

6. Antitubercular _____

7. Macrolide _____

## MATCHING

Match the following drugs with their classes.

_____ 1. Acyclovir      A. Anthelminthic

_____ 2. Mebendazole      B. Antibiotic

_____ 3. Griseofulvin      C. Antituberculin

_____ 4. Keflex      D. Antifungal

_____ 5. Rifampin      E. Antiviral

Copyright © 2007 Elsevier, Inc. All rights reserved.

**RESEARCH ACTIVITY**

1. Access the website *www.cdc.gov*.
   A. What are the latest statistics on HIV/AIDS, TB, and STDs?
   B. Which age group is affected most by each of these diseases?

2. Access the website *http://www.vet.purdue.edu/depts/bms/courses/chmrx/penems.htm*. Read about the many uses of penicillin and its derivatives.

**CRITICAL THINKING**

1. For years medical researchers have been trying to find the cure for the common cold. Why are viruses so difficult to kill? Why does it seem as if they "keep one step ahead" of the researchers?

2. The immune system can be affected by a hectic lifestyle. What are some contributing factors in your lifestyle that might cause your immune system to function below optimum level?

3. HIV/AIDS is a preventable disease. Make a list of measures you can take to avoid contracting the disease.

4. What is the "invincibility factor" in young adults that makes them take risks while thinking, "It'll never happen to me"?

Copyright © 2007 Elsevier, Inc. All rights reserved.

## TERMS AND DEFINITIONS

Select the correct term from the following list and write the corresponding letter in the blank next to the statement.

A. Anaphylactic shock

B. Antigen

C. Bradykinins

D. Dermatitis

E. Erythema

F. Histamine

G. NSAIDs

H. OTC

I. Rhinitis

J. Steroids

K. Systemic

L. Urticaria

M. Vasodilation

_____ 1. Inflammation of the skin associated with itching and burning

_____ 2. Over the counter

_____ 3. A skin eruption of itching wheals

_____ 4. Messenger chemicals produced by the body that help fight inflammation and pain

_____ 5. A substance that interacts with tissues, producing an allergic reaction

_____ 6. A substance that can stimulate an immune response

_____ 7. Pertaining to the whole body rather than to individual body parts

_____ 8. Nonsteroidal antiinflammatory drugs

_____ 9. Chemicals produced by the body that cause inflammation and pain

_____ 10. Redness of the skin, often resulting from capillary dilation

_____ 11. A severe allergic reaction that causes the blood pressure to decrease rapidly, the heart to go into ventricular tachycardia, and the airways to close; a medical emergency that will cause death immediately

_____ 12. Inflammation of the lining of the nose; runny nose

_____ 13. Widening of the blood vessels that allows for increased blood flow

## TRUE OR FALSE

Write T or F next to each statement.

_____ 1. Inflammation is a necessary response for the body to heal itself.

_____ 2. Pain is a response that can be measured scientifically.

_____ 3. Prolonged pain can affect a person's psychological health.

_____ 4. The first company to market aspirin was St. Joseph's.

_____ 5. NSAIDs all work the same, therefore if one brand does not work, neither will another brand.

_____ 6. Steroids have an important role in the maintenance of the body system.

_____ 7. Asthma is a chronic inflammatory disorder.

_____ 8. Antihistamines are used to reduce inflammation and irritation.

_____ 9. Histamine can cause severe migraines.

_____ 10. Most asthma medications are available OTC.

Copyright © 2007 Elsevier, Inc. All rights reserved.

## MULTIPLE CHOICE

Complete each question by circling the best answer.

1. Which of the following is *not* a cause of inflammation?
   A. Infection
   B. Advancing age
   C. Allergy
   D. Injury

2. Which of the following is *not* a symptom of inflammation?
   A. Swelling
   B. Heat
   C. Bleeding
   D. Loss of function in the affected area

3. Aspirin is used to treat
   A. Gout
   B. Inflammation
   C. Fevers
   D. All of the above

4. Aspirin therapy is used to prevent
   A. Stroke
   B. Heart attack
   C. Pulmonary embolism
   D. All of the above

5. Aspirin should not be given to children because its use in that age group has been linked to
   A. Toxic shock syndrome
   B. Reye's syndrome
   C. Chickenpox
   D. Sudden infant death syndrome

6. Which of the following is true about NSAIDs?
   A. All NSAIDs are available in lesser strengths OTC
   B. They are highly addictive
   C. They reduce fever
   D. They increase inflammation

7. Relafen and Toradol are both
   A. NSAIDs
   B. Corticosteroids
   C. Antihistamines
   D. Bronchodilators

8. Asthma attacks can be caused by
   A. Smoking
   B. Stressful situations
   C. A and B
   D. None of the above

9. Which of the following is *not* a side effect of steroidal medications?
   A. Inflammation
   B. Weight gain
   C. Bruising easily
   D. Moon face

10. Which of the following is the only agent considered both an antiasthmatic and an antiallergic agent?
    A. Triamcinolone
    B. Cromolyn sodium
    C. Loratadine
    D. Aspirin

## SHORT ANSWER

1. Explain how the enzyme cyclooxygenase affects the body.

_____

_____

2. What is Reye's syndrome?

_____

_____

3. What three properties do NSAIDs have?

   A. _____
   B. _____
   C. _____

4. What three problems can overuse of NSAIDs cause?

   A. _____
   B. _____
   C. _____

Chapter **25** Antiinflammatories and Antihistamines

Copyright © 2007 Elsevier, Inc. All rights reserved.

5. Name three common types of medications used to treat asthma.

A. _____

B. _____

C. _____

6. What is the difference between a COX-1 inhibitor and a COX-2 inhibitor? _____

_____

_____

## MATCHING

### Matching I
Match the following trade and generic drug names.

_____ 1. Benadryl    A. Albuterol

_____ 2. Azmacort    B. Diphenhydramine

_____ 3. Proventil    C. Celecoxib

_____ 4. Celebrex    D. Naproxen

_____ 5. Anaprox    E. Triamcinolone acetonide

### Matching II
Match the following immune cell responses (see Table 25-1 in text).

_____ 1. Antibodies    A. A globulin found in blood plasma

_____ 2. Leukocytes    B. Large cells that secrete cytokines

_____ 3. Fibrinogen    C. Large type of leukocyte

_____ 4. Monocyte    D. Produced by B lymphocytes

_____ 5. Macrophage    E. White blood cell

## RESEARCH ACTIVITY

1. Access the website *http://medlineplus.gov*.
   A. Make a list of antihistamines available over the counter.
   B. What are the new asthma inhalers available on the market?
   C. Read about insect stings and treatments for them.

2. Access the website *http://www.niaaa.nih.gov/publications/arh23-1/40-54.pdf*. Read about the effects of mixing alcohol with medication.

## CRITICAL THINKING

1. You have just been bitten by a fire ant. Knowing that you are severely allergic to these insect bites, what should be your first course of action to prevent anaphylactic shock?

Copyright © 2007 Elsevier, Inc. All rights reserved.

2. TV advertisements can sometimes be deceiving. Picture this: A man is rowing a boat across a lake, and his arms become sore. He comes over to the dock, where his friend awaits him. The rower complains about his arms, and the friend recommends Tylenol for his sore muscles. What is wrong with this picture?

3. Migraines can be debilitating to the sufferer. When is the best time to take medication for a migraine? What other measures should be taken to reduce the symptoms?

Copyright © 2007 Elsevier, Inc. All rights reserved.

# 26 Vitamins and Minerals

## TERMS AND DEFINITIONS

Select the correct term from the following list and write the corresponding letter in the blank next to the statement.

A. Anemia

B. Avitaminosis

C. Electrolytes

D. Hemoglobin

E. Hypervitaminosis

F. Molecular biosynthesis

G. Intrinsic factor

H. Trace elements

I. Water-soluble vitamins

J. Enzyme

_____ 1. Charged elements, called *cations* (which have a positive charge) and *anions* (which have a negative charge)

_____ 2. Vitamins that are soluble in water and are not readily stored by the body

_____ 3. The making of chemical compounds in a living organism

_____ 4. Vitamin deficiency

_____ 5. The iron-containing blood cell that carries oxygen to the tissues

_____ 6. Elements that are needed by the body in very small amounts

_____ 7. A deficiency of circulating red blood cells; a symptom of disease, not itself a disease

_____ 8. A naturally produced protein necessary for the absorption of vitamin $B_{12}$

_____ 9. A protein that speeds up a reaction by reducing the amount of energy required to initiate the reaction

_____ 10. A condition caused by the presence of too many vitamins; more common with fat-soluble vitamins

## TRUE OR FALSE

Write T or F next to each statement.

_____ 1. Vitamins and minerals are necessary for proper growth and development.

_____ 2. Fat-soluble vitamins are stored in the fat cells of the body.

_____ 3. Vitamin supplements are regulated by the FDA to ensure ingredient safety.

_____ 4. The FDA regulates the recommended daily allowance (RDA) of vitamins and minerals.

_____ 5. All of the B complex vitamins are fat soluble.

_____ 6. Niacin is also known as *nicotine*.

_____ 7. Overcooking vegetables can cause loss of vitamin C.

_____ 8. Minerals are organic substances.

_____ 9. Most of the iron in the body is found in hemoglobin.

_____ 10. Phospholipids are required for cell membrane formation.

Copyright © 2007 Elsevier, Inc. All rights reserved.

## MULTIPLE CHOICE

Complete each question by circling the best answer.

1. Many vitamins and minerals are referred to as
   A. Enzymes
   B. Coenzymes
   C. Antioxidants
   D. Complexes

2. Vitamins A, D, E, and K are all
   A. Water soluble
   B. Fat soluble
   C. Carbohydrates
   D. Minerals

3. A vitamin D deficiency can cause
   A. Blindness
   B. Scurvy
   C. Beriberi
   D. Rickets

4. Vitamin K is responsible for
   A. Blood coagulation factors
   B. Scurvy
   C. Rickets
   D. Lactation

5. All of the B complex vitamins are
   A. Water soluble
   B. Fat soluble
   C. Carbohydrates
   D. Minerals

6. Which of the following is *not* a major function of thiamine?
   A. Carbohydrate metabolism
   B. Energy production
   C. Red blood cell production
   D. Nervous and cardiovascular system well-being

7. Dwarfism, anemia, dementia, depression, and hair loss can all be caused by a deficiency in
   A. Vitamin $B_3$
   B. Vitamin C
   C. Iron
   D. Vitamin $B_{12}$

8. A vitamin C deficiency can cause
   A. Beriberi
   B. Haricari
   C. Rickets
   D. Scurvy

9. Iron deficiency cannot be caused by
   A. Excessive blood loss
   B. Alcoholism
   C. Erythropoietin
   D. Inadequate intestinal absorption

10. An overdose of calcium can cause
    A. Kidney stones
    B. Black stools
    C. Scurvy
    D. Osteoporosis

## FILL IN THE BLANK

1. Trace elements are agents the body requires to run _____ _____.

2. The FDA considers all vitamins, minerals, herbs, amino acids, and extracts _____.

3. Cholecalciferol (vitamin $D_3$) is produced in the skin in the presence of _____.

4. Three drugs that interact with vitamin D are _____, and _____.

5. How does the body produce vitamin K? _____

6. _____ are vitamins that enable proper cellular functioning of the body systems.

7. Three reasons vitamin $B_{12}$ is important for the body are _____, _____, and _____.

8. The main antioxidant vitamins are _____.

9. Iron is important for the transport of _____ in the blood.

10. The most common type of anemia is _____.

Copyright © 2007 Elsevier, Inc. All rights reserved.

## VITAMIN NAMES

Give the chemical names for the following vitamins.

1. Vitamin A   _____

2. Vitamin C   _____

3. Vitamin K   _____

4. Vitamin $B_1$   _____

5. Vitamin $B_{12}$ _____

## CHEMICAL SYMBOLS

Give the chemical symbols for the following minerals.

1. Calcium        _____

2. Chlorine       _____

3. Magnesium   _____

4. Potassium    _____

5. Sodium        _____

6. Iron            _____

7. Zinc            _____

## RESEARCH ACTIVITY

1. Access the website *http://www.sbaa.org/html/sbaa_facts.html*. Answer the following questions:
   A. What causes spina bifida?
   B. What vitamin is important in the prevention of spina bifida?

2. Visit the local health food store or the vitamin section of your local pharmacy.
   A. Make a list of all the types of calcium supplements available.
   B. What are the active ingredients?
   C. What is the recommended daily dose?
   D. Why is it so important to take vitamin D in conjunction with calcium?

3. Access the website *http://www.merck.com/pubs/mmanual/section1/chapter3/3b.htm*. What are the effects of vitamin A deficiency?

## CRITICAL THINKING

1. Have you ever heard of bodybuilders who have vitamin skin odors? Can you really smell like the vitamins you ingest? Explain.

2. Exposure to sunshine activates vitamin D in your body. Does this mean that the more you are exposed to sunshine, the more vitamin D will be activated in your body?

Copyright © 2007 Elsevier, Inc. All rights reserved.

3. Do raw vegetables provide more vitamins than cooked vegetables? Should all vegetables be eaten raw?

4. Most people take vitamins because they feel "run down." Will vitamins really help eliminate that "run down" feeling?

Copyright © 2007 Elsevier, Inc. All rights reserved.

# 27 Vaccines

## TERMS AND DEFINITIONS

Select the correct term from the following list and write the corresponding letter in the blank next to the statement.

A. Acquired immunity

B. Antibodies

C. Antigen

D. Attenuated

E. Globulin

F. Immunity

G. Passive immunity

H. Toxoid

I. Vaccines

_____ 1. The marker on cell surfaces that marks the cell as a "self-cell"; stimulates the production of antibodies

_____ 2. Toxoids or attenuated viral components given to stimulate a response from the body that results in immunity

_____ 3. A type of resistance to infection resulting from an immune response produced by the body or elicited by agents such as vaccines

_____ 4. Immunity acquired through exposure to an antigen or infectious agent

_____ 5. An altered or weakened live vaccine made from the disease organism against which the vaccine is protective

_____ 6. Resistance acquired through a transfer of antibodies from another person, animal, or child

_____ 7. Proteins that are insoluble in water; immune globules protect against disease

_____ 8. Proteins in plasma cells that neutralize or destroy antigens; also known as *immunoglobulins*

_____ 9. A toxin that has been rendered harmless but still invokes an antigen response

## TRUE OR FALSE

Write T or F next to each statement.

_____ 1. The lymphatic system is commonly referred to as the *immune system.*

_____ 2. The thymus node is much larger in children than in adults.

_____ 3. Plasma cells make up a major portion of the body's fighting cells.

_____ 4. Through immunizations, society is better protected against disease.

_____ 5. There are two types of immunity, inactive and passive.

_____ 6. With live vaccines, the risk of full-blown infection is high.

_____ 7. Most vaccines cover either a viral or a bacterial disease that affects humans.

_____ 8. Live virus vaccines must be attenuated before use.

_____ 9. Tetanus vaccine should be given every 6 years for the first 20 years of life.

_____ 10. Vaccines are also available for diseases such as malaria and fungal infections.

_____ 11. The main effect of polio is paralysis of the muscles in the legs and lungs.

_____ 12. If a pregnant mother should contract hepatitis, there is no risk to the fetus.

_____ 13. The primary reason adults get vaccinations is for travel outside the United States.

_____ 14. Pregnant women should not receive a measles vaccine, because it could harm the fetus.

Copyright © 2007 Elsevier, Inc. All rights reserved.

## MULTIPLE CHOICE

Complete each question by circling the best answer.

1. Varicella, MMR, and hepatitis B are all examples of which type of vaccine?
   A. Immune globulin
   B. Antivenins
   C. Viral
   D. Toxoids

2. The larger nodes of the lymphatic system are
   A. Thymus
   B. Tonsils
   C. Spleen
   D. All of the above

3. The primary function of the thymus is to produce
   A. Lymphocytes
   B. Antivenins
   C. Immune globulins
   D. Interferon

4. The function of the spleen is to
   A. Destroy old blood cells
   B. Destroy bacteria and foreign bodies
   C. A and B
   D. None of the above

5. Lymphocytes produce
   A. B cells
   B. T cells
   C. More lymphocytes
   D. Plasma cells
   E. A and B

6. A weakened form of antigen vaccine is given for
   A. Whooping cough
   B. Tetanus

C. Polio
D. All of the above

7. Which of the following is *not* a person at high risk for catching and succumbing to disease?
   A. Chemotherapy patient
   B. Adolescent patient
   C. Transplant patient
   D. AIDS patient

8. Which type of immunity protects from an outside source, such as an immunization vaccine?
   A. Active immunity
   B. Passive immunity
   C. Both A and B
   D. Neither A nor B

9. The vaccines that are required after children start school are
   A. MMR and varicella
   B. Hepatitis B and polio
   C. DPT and HIB
   D. HIB and PCV

10. The vaccine that protects against meningitis is called
    A. Havrix
    B. Varivax
    C. Pneumonococcal polysaccharide
    D. Cytomegalovirus immune globulin

## FILL IN THE BLANK

1. When first contact is made with a foreign body (antigen), _____ are formed.

2. _____ recommends the course of vaccinations for children.

3. _____ occurs when the body is exposed to a disease and actively produces antibodies.

4. Some vaccines are referred to as _____, which are activated _____ toxins.

5. The hepatitis B virus is transmitted through _____ and _____.

6. Another name for *pertussis* is _____; another name for *tetanus* is _____.

7. Mumps affect the _____ glands of the body.

8. The virus that causes chickenpox can also cause _____.

9. Two medications used for shingles are _____ and _____.

10. Immune globulins are attained from a _____ or _____ donor.

11. The only people to receive the anthrax vaccine are the _____.

Copyright © 2007 Elsevier, Inc. All rights reserved.

## MATCHING

Match the following types of vaccines with their sources.

_____ 1. Rabies          A. Viral

_____ 2. Tetanus       B. Immunostimulant

_____ 3. Hepatitis B    C. Toxoid

_____ 4. Etanercept     D. Immunosuppressive

_____ 5. Cyclosporine   E. Antitoxin

## RESEARCH ACTIVITY

1. Access the website *www.cdc.gov*.
   A. What was the latest vaccine released?
   B. How many strains of the hepatitis virus are currently known? How many vaccines are available and to what strain(s)?

2. Access the website *http://www.medformation.com/mf/stayhealthy.nsf/page/immunizechild*. Print the pediatric immunization schedule. How many vaccinations are required for children 0 to 4 years?

3. Access the website *http://www.cdc.gov/nip/recs/adult-schedule.pdf*. Print the adult immunization schedule. How many vaccinations are required for adults?

## CRITICAL THINKING

1. AIDS is a devastating disease. What type of lymphocyte is most important for AIDS patients? Why?

2. In the United States, sanitization and hygiene are stressed, yet people still frequently become ill. Does constant sanitization bring about a healthier immune system or does it weaken it?

Copyright © 2007 Elsevier, Inc. All rights reserved.

3. Botox vaccine is the latest product being used to "reduce or eliminate wrinkles." Can repeated Botox injections harm the recipients or cause them to build up a resistance to the toxin?

4. The World Health Organization (WHO) has been working tirelessly to eradicate infectious diseases throughout the world, with much success. What would happen to the planet's population if all infectious diseases were eradicated and vaccinations were not needed?

Copyright © 2007 Elsevier, Inc. All rights reserved.

# 28 Oncology Agents

## TERMS AND DEFINITIONS

Select the correct term from the following list and write the corresponding letter in the blank next to the statement.

A. Antineoplastic

B. Benign

C. Biopsy

D. Cancer

E. Carcinogen

F. Chemotherapy

G. DNA

H. Invasive

I. Leukemia

J. Lymphoma

K. Malignant

L. Melanoma

M. Metastasis

N. Mitosis

O. Morphology

P. Mutation

Q. Neoplasm

R. Oncogene

S. Remission

T. Sarcoma

_____ 1. A previously normal gene that may be adversely affected by an infection, such as a retrovirus, that causes a mutation and may produce cancer

_____ 2. A procedure in which a piece of tissue is removed from a patient for examination and diagnosis

_____ 3. The appearance of an organism, such as its size, shape, and characteristics

_____ 4. The treatment of a disease with toxic chemicals to slow the progress of the disease or to kill cells

_____ 5. A malignant neoplasm of the pigmented cells of the skin; may metastasize to other organs

_____ 6. A progressive disease marked by malignancy of the blood-forming cells in the hemopoietic tissues and organs and the bloodstream, resulting in the circulation of abnormal blood cells

_____ 7. A general term used to describe malignant neoplasms

_____ 8. An abnormal tissue growth

_____ 9. The tendency of a tumor or mass to move into nearby tissues or organs or both

_____ 10. A nonmalignant neoplasm

_____ 11. The complex nucleic acids that are bases for genetic continuance

_____ 12. The movement or spread of cancerous cells through the body to organs in distant areas

_____ 13. The span of time during which a disease such as cancer is not spreading; may be permanent or temporary

_____ 14. Cellular reproduction that creates two identical daughter cells from the parent cells' DNA

_____ 15. A substance or chemical that can increase a person's risk of developing cancer

_____ 16. An invasive, destructive pattern of rapid, abnormal cell growth that is often fatal

_____ 17. An unexpected change in the molecular structure within the DNA that causes a permanent change in cells

Copyright © 2007 Elsevier, Inc. All rights reserved.

____ 18. A malignant neoplastic growth arising from connective tissue

____ 19. An agent used to prevent the development, proliferation, or growth of neoplastic cells

____ 20. A term used to describe a malignant disorder of lymphoid tissue

## TRUE OR FALSE

Write T or F next to each statement

____ 1. If a person has cancer, it certainly means death.

____ 2. Cancer can strike any area of the body.

____ 3. Benign tumors are cancerous.

____ 4. Cancer can be caused by environmental contaminants.

____ 5. If cancer is diagnosed in the early stages, it may be surgically removed.

____ 6. Fewer than 100 known cancers plague the human body.

____ 7. Kaposi's sarcoma is a type of cancer that affects the skin.

____ 8. The risk of cancer declines as a person ages beyond 65 years.

____ 9. Children tend to respond to chemotherapy and to recuperate more quickly than older adults.

____ 10. Chemotherapeutic agents destroy healthy cells along with cancer cells.

## MULTIPLE CHOICE

Complete each question by circling the best answer.

1. Which of the following is *not* a form that can turn into a malignant or cancerous tumor?
   A. Pimples
   B. Moles
   C. Warts
   D. Lesions

2. Which of the following is *not* a type of cancer?
   A. Carcinoma
   B. Leukemia
   C. Lymphoma
   D. Glioma

3. Some types of cancer-causing agents include
   A. Radioactive materials
   B. Coal
   C. Dyes
   D. All of the above

4. Which of the following is *not* a means by which cancers can be identified and treated?
   A. MRIs
   B. EKGs
   C. Sonograms
   D. Biopsies

5. Breast and prostate cancers are being cured more often as a result of
   A. Checkups
   B. Vaccines
   C. A and B
   D. None of the above

6. Leukemia arises in the
   A. Bone marrow
   B. Lymphatic system
   C. A and B
   D. None of the above

7. Treatments for cancer include all of the following *except*
   A. Surgery
   B. Radiation
   C. Vitamins
   D. Chemotherapy

8. Cytarabine, fluorouracil, and methotrexate are
   A. Mitotic inhibitors
   B. Antibiotics
   C. Alkylating agents
   D. Antimetabolites

9. Nitrogen mustards were first used in
   A. The Vietnam War
   B. The Korean War
   C. World War I
   D. World War II

10. A nuclear pharmacy technician must wear a
    A. Badge stating that the person is a nuclear technician
    B. Radioactive meter
    C. Lead apron
    D. All of the above

**114**

Copyright © 2007 Elsevier, Inc. All rights reserved.

## FILL IN THE BLANK

1. _____ lymphoma is a cancer of the lymphatic cell located in the lymph node.

2. Most treatments for cancer include more than one _____ and may be followed up with or preceded by _____ therapy.

3. In cancer treatment, radiation is classified by the _____ of the rays. Alpha and beta rays are used to treat _____ lesions, whereas gamma rays are used to treat _____ lesions.

4. Antimetabolites are often used in the treatment of _____.

5. Side effects of antibiotics used in cancer treatment include _____, _____, _____, _____, and _____.

6. Vinblastine and vincristine are _____ derived from plants.

7. Two major types of alkylating agents are _____ and _____.

8. _____ are agents that cross the blood-brain barrier and that can be used to treat _____ cancer.

9. Two main biologic response modifiers used to treat side effects of chemotherapy are _____ and _____.

10. Agents used in nuclear pharmacy are called _____.

## MATCHING

**Matching I**
Match the following drugs with their classification.

| | |
|---|---|
| _____ 1. Bleomycin | A. Alkylating agent |
| _____ 2. Cyclophosphamide | B. Hormone |
| _____ 3. Methotrexate | C. Antimitotic |
| _____ 4. Vinblastine | D. Antibiotic |
| _____ 5. Topotecan | E. Antimetabolite |

**Matching II**
Match the following drugs with their indications.

| | |
|---|---|
| _____ 1. Vinorelbine | A. Myelocytic leukemia |
| _____ 2. Paclitaxel | B. Testicular cancer |
| _____ 3. Cytarabine | C. Lung cancer |
| _____ 4. Dactinomycin | D. Ovarian/breast cancer |
| _____ 5. Ifosfamide | E. Wilms' tumor |

## RESEARCH ACTIVITY

1. Access the website *www.cancerguide.org*. Take the tour of the website to see what kind of information is offered.

2. Access the website *www.cancer.gov*. Choose the section Statistics. Choose two types of cancers and get the latest statistics on them.

3. Access the website *http://www.cancerquest.org/index.cfm?page=183*. List the various types of cancer treatments discussed.

4. Can a known poison be used to treat cancer? Access the website *http://www.hon.ch/News/HSN/512218.html* to see.

Copyright © 2007 Elsevier, Inc. All rights reserved.

1. A woman poses this question to her doctor: "My grandmother, aunt, and cousin all died of breast cancer. Does it mean that I will get cancer, too?"
   A. Is cancer hereditary?
   B. Should the woman be thinking about a mastectomy, even if she does not currently have cancer?

2. Many scientists claim that the cure for cancer lies in the plants of the world's great forests. These forests are disappearing as a result of the growth in the world's population and the use of land to mine for gold or to grow food. Should governments get involved in plant-targeted cancer research? What can be done to foster research in this area?

3. Tobacco is a known carcinogen, yet people still use it. What would you use to illustrate the devastating effects of tobacco on the respiratory system?

Copyright © 2007 Elsevier, Inc. All rights reserved.

# 29 Microbiology

## TERMS AND DEFINITIONS

Select the correct term from the following list and write the corresponding letter in the blank next to the statement.

A. Aerobic

B. Anaerobic

C. Binary fusion

D. Biology

E. Catalyst

F. Enzyme

G. Facultative anaerobe

H. Heterotrophic

I. Microbial

J. Microbiology

K. Morphology

L. Peptidoglycan

M. Species

N. Taxonomy

O. Vectors

P. Virology

Q. Virus

_____ 1. The host that carries the disease; does not need to be living

_____ 2. The method of reproduction by which a single cell divides into two separate cells

_____ 3. The substance that comprises bacterial cell walls are specifically of Gram-positive and Gram-negative microbes

_____ 4. A protein that causes chemical changes to take place

_____ 5. Refers to microorganisms not visible without a microscope

_____ 6. Organisms that need air to survive

_____ 7. An organism that replicates using the host's cell parts, including DNA, ribosomes, and proteins

_____ 8. A term of Latin origin meaning "kind"

_____ 9. A molecule that allows chemical reactions to take place rapidly but is not altered in the reaction

_____ 10. The ability to reproduce asexually

_____ 11. Organisms that live in the absence of oxygen

_____ 12. The study of microscopic organisms

_____ 13. The study of viruses

_____ 14. A microorganism that can live with or without oxygen

_____ 15. The science of the classification and nomenclature of organisms

_____ 16. The study of life

_____ 17. The study of characteristics of organisms

## TRUE OR FALSE

Write T or F next to each statement.

_____ 1. Viruses are smaller than bacteria.

_____ 2. Louis Pasteur's lifetime was called the golden age of biology.

_____ 3. The study of naming and classifying organisms is called *taxidermy*.

_____ 4. Viruses are not included in the five kingdoms.

_____ 5. Plants acquire energy differently from animals.

_____ 6. Many diseases are transmitted easily by plants.

**117**

Copyright © 2007 Elsevier, Inc. All rights reserved.

_____ 7. Animal cells get their energy from food rather than from sunlight.

_____ 8. Vectors are the carriers of organisms.

_____ 9. Algae do not need light to survive.

_____ 10. Humans are more susceptible to fungal infections than are plants.

## MULTIPLE CHOICE

Complete each question by circling the best answer.

1. The study of microbiology includes all of the following *except*
   A. Bacteria
   B. Fungi
   C. Protists
   D. All of the above

2. The first microscope was invented by
   A. Gregory Hacker
   B. Herbert Ritchie
   C. Robert Hooke
   D. Steven Martin

3. It was believed that flies came from
   A. Manure
   B. Decaying corpses
   C. Snakes
   D. All of the above

4. Louis Pasteur proved that
   A. Unseen microorganisms exist in the air
   B. DNA is a genetic material
   C. Cleaning the hands between surgeries reduces the spread of infection
   D. All of the above

5. The plant kingdom includes all of the following *except*
   A. Mosses
   B. Viruses
   C. Ferns
   D. Conifers

6. Plants have chloroplasts, which are used to
   A. Convert sunlight to energy
   B. Convert sunlight to fragrance
   C. Convert energy to fragrance
   D. Convert fragrance to energy

7. Which of the following is *not* a way people benefit from plants?
   A. Food
   B. Clothing
   C. Touch
   D. Building materials

8. Which of the following is *not* an example of a complex animal organism?
   A. Frog
   B. Sponge
   C. Kangaroo
   D. Spider

9. Dysentery is spread by transfer from
   A. Penis to cervix
   B. Cervix to penis
   C. Mouth to penis
   D. Feces to mouth

10. Conditions caused by a fungus are
    A. Athlete's foot
    B. Sepsis
    C. Vaginal infections
    D. All of the above

## FILL IN THE BLANK

1. One difference between eukaryotes and prokaryotes is that eukaryotes have a _____ and prokaryotes do not.

2. Digoxin is taken from the _____ plant and is used to treat _____ conditions.

3. *Trichomonas vaginalis* is a _____ that causes infection in the male _____ and in the _____ of females.

4. The fungi kingdom is divided into _____ fungi and _____ _____.

5. _____ are responsible for decomposing plant organisms.

6. *Candida albicans* is part of _____ _____ in the mouth and genitourinary tract of humans.

7. Penicillin destroys _____ by interacting with _____ present in the cell walls of bacteria.

8. _____ destroy bacteria by breaking down their cell walls.

9. The enzyme that renders penicillins useless against bacteria is _____.

10. Narrow-spectrum antibiotics affect _____ _____ microbes, and broad-spectrum antibiotics affect _____ _____ microbes.

Copyright © 2007 Elsevier, Inc. All rights reserved.

## SHORT ANSWER

1. How are viruses classified? _____

_____

2. How do viruses survive? _____

_____

3. How are viruses identified? _____

_____

4. How does the drug zidovudine work? _____

_____

## GRAM STAIN LAB PROCEDURE

This practice exercise is a step-by-step procedure for performing a Gram stain (see Chapter 29 in the text). It can help you to gain confidence in viewing organisms through a microscope and to understand the purpose of the staining process.

### Materials Needed

Glass slide
Small tongs or large tweezers
Marker
Square plastic slide cover
Toothpicks

Iodine dropper bottle
Violet dropper bottle
Water dropper bottle
Long lighter
Microscope

### Step-by-Step Procedure

1. Draw a circle on the underside of the glass side (the topside will hold the sample).

2. Lightly scrape the inside of your cheek with the toothpick.

3. Scrape the toothpick onto the top of the glass slide (the side not marked with the circle).

4. Use tongs or tweezers to hold the slide at the edge. Wave the lighter back and forth quickly three times under the slide; this sets the cells onto the slide.

5. Over a sink or pan, apply the solutions.

6. Place one drop of iodine. Wait 1 minute, then rinse with water.

7. Place one drop of violet. Wait 1 minute, then rinse with water.

8. Place the plastic slide cover over the sample and view the sample under the microscope.

9. First view at 10×; draw what you see.

10. Now view at 40×; draw what you see.

### Safety Tips

1. When using anything glass, always handle the article extremely carefully, to avoid breaking it or injuring yourself with an intact or a broken item.

2. If glass breaks, clean up and dispose of the item according to institutional procedures.

3. Use caution when scraping the inside of your cheek with the toothpick. Do not poke your cheek, because this can cause injury.

4. Be extremely careful when using an open flame; do not leave it unattended.

5. Always wipe the eyepieces of the microscope with alcohol before and after using the instrument to reduce the chance of spreading infection.

**119**

Copyright © 2007 Elsevier, Inc. All rights reserved.

## MATCHING

Match the microbes with the correct disease or condition.

_____ 1. Protozoon      A. HIV

_____ 2. Bacterium      B. Roundworms

_____ 3. Virus      C. Malaria

_____ 4. Helminth      D. Ringworm

_____ 5. Fungus      E. Meningitis

## RESEARCH ACTIVITY

1. Access the website _http://co.howard.in.us/health/insect.htm_ and learn about vectors of disease.

2. Access the website _http://poisonivy.aesir.com/_ and learn facts about poison ivy and poison oak.

3. Access the website _http://www.cdc.gov/ncidod/eid/vol4no3/falkow.htm._ Who speaks for the microbes?

## CRITICAL THINKING

1. If you had the chance to do an educational presentation on HIV/AIDS, what five things would you stress the most in your presentation?

2. Many companies market antibacterial soaps, cleansers, and so forth. What would be the result of overuse of these products?

3. Handwashing is one of the most important tools for universal precautions and for preventing the spread of germs. What tool can you use to convince children and adults to teach about the importance of handwashing?

**120**

Copyright © 2007 Elsevier, Inc. All rights reserved.

# 30 Chemistry

## TERMS AND DEFINITIONS

Select the correct term from the following list and write the corresponding letter in the blank next to the statement.

A. Amino acids

B. Anabolism

C. Atom

D. Atomic mass

E. Catabolism

F. Covalent bond

G. Electron

H. Enzyme

I. Gram

J. Kcal

K. Ion

L. Ionic bond

M. Macro

N. Metabolism

O. Meter

P. Micro

Q. Mole

R. Molecule

S. Neutron

T. Nucleic acid

U. Orbit

V. Proton

W. Valence

_____ 1. The smallest unit of an element

_____ 2. The sharing of electrons between two atoms

_____ 3. A basic unit of weight of the metric system equal to the weight of a cubic centimeter or a milliliter of water; 1000 mg

_____ 4. The transfer of electrons between two atoms

_____ 5. The basic measurement of length in the metric system

_____ 6. A subset of an atom that does not contain a charge

_____ 7. A subatomic particle of an atom that holds a positive charge

_____ 8. The bases contained within deoxyribonucleic acid (DNA)

_____ 9. Large

_____ 10. A protein that helps a reaction take place in a living organism without changing chemical enzymes

_____ 11. The mass of an atom expressed in the units of $1.660 \times 10^{-24}$

_____ 12. To break down; the destruction phase of metabolism

_____ 13. A measurement of energy or heat expended or used up in a chemical activity

_____ 14. Small

_____ 15. The rotation of electrons around the atom

_____ 16. Avogadro's number; $6.02 \times 10^{23}$ atoms, molecules, or ions

_____ 17. The smallest subset of an atom that contains a negative charge

_____ 18. An atom or group of atoms with a leftover unbalanced charge

_____ 19. Macromolecules that make up proteins

_____ 20. The physical and chemical change that takes place within an organism

_____ 21. The smallest particle of a compound

_____ 22. The number of electrons gained, lost, or shared when an atom bonds with another atom

_____ 23. To build up; the construction phase of metabolism

**121**

Copyright © 2007 Elsevier, Inc. All rights reserved.

## TRUE OR FALSE

Write T or F next to each statement.

_____ 1. Chemistry has little to do with the health care field.

_____ 2. Chemistry uses many of the same metric terms as pharmacy.

_____ 3. Subatomic particles are the smallest units known to humans.

_____ 4. Chemical reactions make life happen.

_____ 5. The human body needs nutrients on a monthly basis.

_____ 6. Aminoglycosides can build up in the kidneys.

_____ 7. To ensure sterility, a new TPN must be hung every week.

_____ 8. Each TPN is tailor-made to the patient's specific needs.

_____ 9. Copper is a metal the body uses in minute amounts.

_____ 10. Iodine is needed for proper functioning of the kidney.

## MULTIPLE CHOICE

Complete each question by circling the best answer.

1. Each atom has the same number of protons and electrons, therefore it is
   A. Positive
   B. Negative
   C. Neutral
   D. None of the above

2. Organic chemistry is the study of
   A. Substances that contain carbon
   B. Substances that contain dioxide
   C. Substances that contain oxygen
   D. All of the above

3. Enzymes are composed of elements that can cause
   A. A reaction
   B. A faster reaction
   C. A reaction to stop
   D. All of the above

4. Which patient will *not* require a TPN?
   A. A patient who will not eat food
   B. A comatose patient
   C. A patient healing from stomach surgery
   D. All of the above

5. Zinc is needed in
   A. Large amounts
   B. Very minute amounts
   C. A and B
   D. None of the above

6. When amino acids join together, they cause
   A. Dehydration
   B. Proteins to be made
   C. Nausea and vomiting
   D. Diarrhea

7. Metabolism is necessary for the control of
   A. Hormones
   B. Protein synthesis
   C. pH, fat, and glucose levels
   D. All of the above

8. Neutrons are
   A. Positively charged
   B. Negatively charged
   C. Not charged
   D. A and B

9. Which of the following are made by joining two or more atoms?
   A. Carbohydrates
   B. Lipids
   C. Proteins
   D. All of the above

10. The smallest part of an element is a (an)
   A. Atom
   B. Molecule
   C. Proton
   D. Neutron

## SHORT ANSWER

1. How is the salt NaCl used in the hospital? _____

_____

2. Inorganic chemistry studies _____ _____

_____. Organic chemistry studies

_____

3. What is the purpose of lab tests? _____

_____

Copyright © 2007 Elsevier, Inc. All rights reserved.

4. The ingredients of a hyperal (TPN) bag include _____,
_____, and _____.

5. Where is phosphorus found in the body, and what enzyme does it help to make? _____
_____

6. What is the range of the pH scale, and what is the normal pH range of the blood? _____
_____

7. How many main amino acids are there and for what are they used? _____
_____

## FILL IN THE BLANK

1. The two types of bonding between atoms are _____ and _____.

2. The _____ _____ of elements has all the known elements strategically placed according to their properties.

3. The metal _____ by itself is highly reactive and would explode if it came in contact with oxygen.

4. Hydrogen peroxide is used as an _____ in households.

5. The human body is able to produce energy and perform other functions quickly because of _____.

## CHEMICAL COMPOUNDS

Give the formula for the following chemical compounds.

1. Water _____

2. Ferrous sulfate _____

3. Sodium chloride _____

4. Potassium chloride _____

5. Hydrochloric acid _____

6. Sodium bicarbonate _____

## RESEARCH ACTIVITY

1. Access the website *http://www.madsci.org/posts/archives/dec98/912791455.Mb.r.html*. What is the chemical makeup of the human body?

2. Access the website *http://www.nyu.edu/pages/mathmol/library/drugs/index.html*. Look at the chemical structures for the various drugs.

Copyright © 2007 Elsevier, Inc. All rights reserved.

## CRITICAL THINKING

1. You went out on Friday night for pizza and a movie with friends. During the course of the evening, in addition to pizza, you ate popcorn and candy and drank soda. By the end of the night you were extremely thirsty. What chemical compounds in the pizza, popcorn, and soda contributed to your thirst?

2. Is ammonia ($NH_4$), a byproduct produced in the body, the same type of ammonia you can buy in the grocery store?

3. If you were to market a drink that contained all the chemicals the body needs, what would your ingredients be?

Copyright © 2007 Elsevier, Inc. All rights reserved.

**CHAPTER 2 LAB SHEET**

State whether the following are C-I, C-II, C-III, C-IV, or C-V drugs. Provide examples as needed.

1. Drugs with acceptable medicinal use but a high potential for abuse, including severe psychological or physical dependence: _____

   Give two examples.

   A. _____

   B. _____

2. Drugs with no acceptable medicinal use in the United States, high potential for abuse, and lack of accepted safety for use under medical supervision: _____

   Give two examples.

   A. _____

   B. _____

3. Give an example of a drug that is classified both as a C-II and a C-III drug. _____

4. Give two examples of C-IV drugs.

   A. _____

   B. _____

5. An example of a C-V drug is _____.

6. Some C-V drugs are dispensed without a prescription. State four requirements that must be met.

   A. _____

   B. _____

   C. _____

   D. _____

7. Prescription labels for C-II, C-III, C-IV, and C-V drugs must have the following:

   A. _____

   B. _____

   C. _____

   D. _____

   E. _____

   F. _____

8. How do you verify a DEA number?

   _____

9. What auxiliary label must be put on all prescription labels for C-II, C-III, and C-IV drugs?

   _____

   _____

Copyright © 2007 Elsevier, Inc. All rights reserved.

## Metric Conversion Quiz

1. 56 mL = _____ L

2. 2,346,097 mcg = _____ g

3. 84 kg = _____ mg

4. 234 L = _____ mL

5. 986 g = _____ kg

6. 34,587 mg = _____ g

7. 324 g = _____ mcg

8. 2,900,867 mcg = _____ kg

9. 876 mL = _____ L

10. 68.76 kg = _____ mg

11. 235.98 mL = _____ L

12. 0.678 L = _____ mL

13. 0.586 g = _____ mg

14. 0.00367 g = _____ mcg

15. 0.56 L = _____ mL

16. 879 kg = _____ mcg

17. 119 mcg = _____ mg

18. Four tenths of a milligram = _____ mcg

19. Five thousandths of a gram = _____ mg

20. Two and six tenths liters = _____ mL

21. Four and two tenths grams = _____ mg

22. 50 kg = _____ mg

23. 2,703,000 mcg = _____ g

24. 9,875 mL = _____ L

25. 89 L = _____ mcL

## Prescription Calculations

Calculate the number of tablets or capsules needed for each prescription.

1. Choledyl 400 mg bid × 15 days _____

2. Slow-K tid × 30 days_____

3. Synthroid 25 mcg qd × 60 days _____

4. Tetracycline 500 mg qid × 60 days _____

5. Ampicillin 250 mg tid × 12 days _____

6. Diamox 500 mg bid × 90 days _____

7. Prednisone 10 mg 2 tid × 5 days, 2 bid × 3 days, then 1 bid × 3 days, 1 qd × 2 days, 1 qd × 1 day, and then stop
   _____

Copyright © 2007 Elsevier, Inc. All rights reserved.

1. You have been given five vials. Identify the following from the vial labels.
   A. Trade and generic drug names
   B. Strength of the medication
   C. NDC number or bar code number
   D. Lot number or control number
   E. Expiration date

   Use a blank sheet of paper to record your findings. Use the following format for each vial.
   Vial number _____

   A. _____

   B. _____

   C. _____

   D. _____

   E. _____

2. Interpret the following prescriptions. Write your answer in a complete sentence. Use the following "key words": take, instill, place, inject, insert.
   A. 1 tsp PCN PO qid × 10 days
   _____

   B. 2 gtt Pilocar OU bid
   _____

   C. 3 caps Pancrease PO tid ac
   _____

   D. 1 supp pr qhs × 3 days
   _____

   E. 10 mg MS IM prn pain
   _____

   F. 1 tab sl for chest pain
   _____

   G. 2 tabs Phenergan PO prn N&V
   _____

   H. 250 mg TCN cap tid PO c̄ meals for acne
   _____

   I. 30 mL MOM PO ac and hs prn
   _____

   J. ut. Dict cream
   _____

## Interpretation Exercise A

Interpret the following prescriptions. Write your answer in a complete sentence.

1. Maalox 30 cc 1 hr ac and pc and hs
   _____

2. Ecotrin 325 mg qam
   _____

3. ASA 650 mg q4-6h prn pain
   _____

4. Phenergan 25 mg IM q4-5h prn N&V
   _____

Copyright © 2007 Elsevier, Inc. All rights reserved.

5. NTG 0.4 mg sl prn chest pain

_____

6. Amphojel 30 cc tid ac and 15 cc prn

_____

7. Amoxicillin susp 1 tsp tid

_____

8. Vitamin K inj 10 mg IM or SQ qwk

_____

9. ≠ Lasix to 80 mg PO tid

_____

10. MS 4 mg IV in RR

_____

11. MOM 1 oz hs prn

_____

12. PCN 2 cap qid × 10 d

_____

13. 2 gtt OS bid

_____

14. 1 gtt al qd ac swimming

_____

15. 1 supp pr qhs × 3 d

_____

## Interpretation Exercise B

Interpret the following prescriptions. Write your answer in a complete sentence.

1. 2 tabs PO tid

_____

2. 1 tbsp PO bid

_____

3. 1 gtt au qd

_____

4. 3 caps PO ac for ha

_____

5. 1 cap PO ac and pc

_____

6. Bacitracin ud dict

_____

7. 2 Tylenol 325 mg PO bid for pain

_____

8. 10 mg MS IM q6h prn

_____

Copyright © 2007 Elsevier, Inc. All rights reserved.

**Weekly Journal Article**

The students should evaluate the presentations of classmates.

1. Choose a pharmacy journal.

2. Read one article that interests you.

3. Be prepared to discuss that article in the next lab. Be able to answer the following questions:
   A. What are the title and subject of the article?
   B. Who is the author?
   C. What is the subject of the article?
   D. What did you learn from this article?

## CHAPTER 8 LAB SHEET

**Prescription Interpretation**

1. Interpret the following outpatient script.

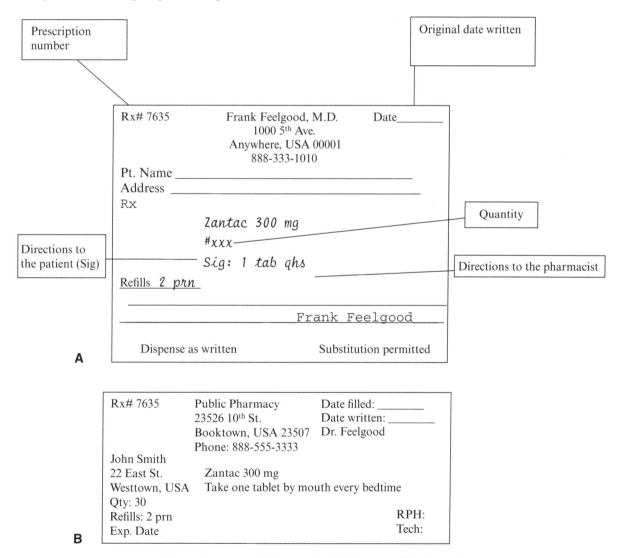

**A,** Outpatient prescription sample. **B,** Pharmacy label sample.

Copyright © 2007 Elsevier, Inc. All rights reserved.

```
Rx# 1232              Frank Feelgood, M.D.        Date _____
                          1000 5th Ave.
                        Anywhere, USA 00001
                          888-333-1010
Pt. Name _____
Address _____
Rx
        Augmentin 125 mg/5 ml Oral Susp.
        #150 cc
        Sig: 1 tsp po tid × 10 days
Refills  0
_____           Frank Feelgood

Dispense as written            Substitution permitted
```

A. Name the drug and give its strength. _____

B. What are the directions to the pharmacist? _____

_____

C. Write the directions to the patient in a complete sentence. _____

_____

D. Are there any refills? _____

2. Interpret the following outpatient script.

```
Rx# 1232              Frank Feelgood, M.D.        Date _____
                          1000 5th Ave.
                        Anywhere, USA 00001
                          888-333-1010
Pt. Name _____
Address _____
Rx
        Ceftin 250 mg
        #20
        Sig: 1 tab po bid
Refills  0
_____           Frank Feelgood

Dispense as written            Substitution permitted
```

A. Name the drug and give its strength. _____

B. What are the directions to the pharmacist? _____

_____

C. Write the directions to the patient in a complete sentence. _____

_____

D. Are there any refills? _____

E. Will you dispense a trade or generic drug? _____

                    Copyright © 2007 Elsevier, Inc. All rights reserved.

3. Interpret the following outpatient script.

```
┌─────────────────────────────────────────────────────────────┐
│  Rx# 1232          Frank Feelgood, M.D.    Date _____       │
│                         1000 5ᵗʰ Ave.       DEA# AF264311      │
│                       Anywhere, USA 00001                     │
│                         888-333-1010                          │
│  Pt. Name _____             │
│  Address _____               │
│  Rx                                                           │
│                   Tylenol #3                                  │
│                   #10                                         │
│                   Sig: 1 tab po q4-6h   prn pain              │
│  Refills                                                      │
│  _____        Frank Feelgood____              │
│                                                               │
│     Dispense as written         Substitution permitted        │
│                                                               │
└─────────────────────────────────────────────────────────────┘
```

A. Name the drug and give its strength. _____

B. What are the directions to the pharmacist? _____

_____

C. Write the directions to the patient in a complete sentence. _____

_____

D. Are there any refills? _____

E. Use the DEA calculation formula to determine whether this is a true DEA number. Show your work.

_____

**Community Prescription Filling Exercise**

Objective: To select the appropriate drug from the shelf and fill it according to the physician's directions.

1. Select the appropriate drug and confirm its name and strength.

2. Determine the quantity necessary according to the prescription directions.

3. Is the necessary quantity available?

4. Select the appropriate container size.

5. Prepare a label, following state requirements.

6. Count out the drug using counting trays.

7. Determine what auxiliary labels are necessary.

8. Present the final product to be checked by the RPh (always have stock vial with prepared product).

9. Do not forget to initial where necessary.

Copyright © 2007 Elsevier, Inc. All rights reserved.

Inpatient Pharmacy

Community Hospital, Inc.

Patient Name: _____

Acct.# _____

Room# _____ Floor_____

PHYSICIAN'S ORDER SHEET

DRUG ALLERGIES: penicillin

| Date and Time | RN Signature | Order begin here: |
|---|---|---|
| 7/25/03 | | Elavil 25 mg po stat x 1 |
| 8:00 am | | Elavil 50 mg po qhs |
| | | Dulcolax supp. x 1 |
| | | Dr. Feelgood |
| | 8:30 AM | |
| | MLamb | |
| 7/25/03 | | Balance diet as tolerated |
| | | If no response to Dulcolax give MOM 30 cc today |
| | | Please remove remainder of staples |
| | LSmith | Dr. Feelgood |
| | | |
| | | |
| | | |
| | | |

## Interpretation Exercise A

Refer to the preceding order.

1. List all the medications ordered with their corresponding directions and quantities.

A. _____

_____

B. _____

_____

C. _____

_____

 Copyright © 2007 Elsevier, Inc. All rights reserved.

D. _____

_____

2. Are there any allergies? If yes, what are they? _____

_____

Community Hospital, Inc.

Patient Name: _____

Acct.# _____

Room# _____ Floor_____

PHYSICIAN'S ORDER SHEET

DRUG ALLERGIES:

| Date and Time | RN Signature | Order begin here: |
|---|---|---|
| 8/01/03 | | Postop orders: |
| 9:00 am | | 1) vs in RR, then q6h |
| | | 2) I&O q4h |
| | | 3) Foley cath |
| | | 4) Strict bed rest |
| | | 5) Low-residue diet |
| | | 6) IV D5 1/2NS @75 cc/hr + 30 mEq KCl |
| | | 7) MSO$_4$ 10 mg IM Q3h prn severe pain |
| | | 8) Percocet 1 po q4h prn moderate pain |
| | | 9) Ativan 1 mg IV q6h |
| | | 10) Phenergan 25 mg IM or po q4h prn N&V |
| | | 11) Heparin 5000 u sc bid |
| | | 12) TED hose full length |
| | | 13) Tenormin 50 mg po qd |
| | | 14) Dyazide 1 po qd |
| | | 15) Courtesy notification Dr. Jim Bean/ Dr. John Page |

**Interpretation Exercise B**

1. Discuss the preceding physician's order.

_____

_____

_____

2. Identify all medication orders pertaining to pharmacy.

_____

_____

_____

Copyright © 2007 Elsevier, Inc. All rights reserved.

## Oral Liquid Exercise

Objective: To select and retrieve the appropriate liquid from the shelf, calculate the correct dose, and prepare and label the product correctly.

1. Select the appropriate liquid.

2. Identify the concentration of the liquid.

3. Observe what type of liquid it is (e.g., solution, syrup).

4. Calculate the necessary dosage according to the medication order.

5. Prepare the liquid in an oral syringe.

6. Label the product correctly.

7. Present the final product to be checked by the RPh.

| Name of Drug | Concentration | Dose Required | #mL (calc) |
|---|---|---|---|
| 1. Hydroxyzine | (10 mg/5 mL) | Dose: 5 mg | |
| 2. Duphalac | (10 g/15 mL) | Dose: 7.5 g | |
| 3. Ephedrine sulfate | (4 mg/1 mL) | Dose: 4 mg | |
| 4. Mestinon | (60 mg/5 mL) | Dose: 75 mg | |
| 5. Retrovir | (50 mg/5 mL) | Dose: 40 mg | |
| 6. Kaon | (20 mEq/15 mL) | Dose: 10 mEq | |
| 7. Alupent | (10 mg/5 mL) | Dose: 12 mg | |
| 8. Modane | (37.5 mg/5 mL) | Dose: 25 mg | |
| 9. Neo-Calglucon | (1.8 g/5 mL) | Dose: 2 g | |
| 10. Dexamethasone | (0.5 mg/0.5 mL) | Dose: 0.8 mg | |
| 11. Diphenhydramine | (12.5 mg/5 mL) | Dose: 10 mg | |
| 12. NegGram | (250 mg/5 mL) | Dose: 750 mg | |
| 13. Symmetrel | (50 mg/5 mL) | Dose: 30 mg | |
| 14. Vistaril | (25 mg/5 mL) | Dose: 30 mg | |

Copyright © 2007 Elsevier, Inc. All rights reserved.

## Compounding Ointments

### Materials
Ointment slab
Spatula
28 g petrolatum (Vaseline)
2 g boric acid
1 drop food coloring

### Procedure
1. Weigh out the Vaseline.
2. Weigh out the boric acid.
3. Place the Vaseline on the ointment slab.
4. Spread it with the spatula.
5. Add the boric acid and work it into the Vaseline.
6. After the boric acid has been incorporated into the Vaseline, add a drop of food coloring.
7. Work the food coloring into the Vaseline.
8. Place this prepared ointment in the ointment jar.
9. Affix the prepared label.
10. Place the final product on the counter to be checked.

## Punch Method Capsule Preparation

### Materials
4 oz cornstarch
10 empty capsules
Paper towels
Class A prescription balance or electronic balance

### Procedure
1. Place 4 oz of cornstarch on the paper towels on a flat surface.
2. Pull apart a capsule.
3. Repeatedly punch the bottom half of the capsule into the cornstarch until the capsule is filled.
4. Cover the capsule with the remaining half.
5. Clean off the capsule with a paper towel.
6. Fill all the capsules using this punch method.
7. Weigh each capsule and ensure that all 10 capsules weigh within 0.05 mg of each other.

Copyright © 2007 Elsevier, Inc. All rights reserved.

## IV Calculations

1. An order is written for a 60 mg Lasix injection. A stock bottle of Lasix is 20 mg/mL.

    A. How many milliliters of Lasix are required to fill this order? _____

2. An order is written for 30 mEq KCl in 1 L D5% 1/2 NS q8h. Run IVF at 125 mL/hr.

    A. What is D5% 1/2 NS? _____

    B. Is this an LVP? _____

    C. The concentration of KCl is 2 mEq/mL. How many milliliters are needed for this order?

    _____

    D. How long should one bag last? _____

    E. How many bags are necessary for a 24-hour period? _____

3. An order reads: Ancef 1 g in D5% 100 mL to be used as a preop; 10 mL are used to reconstitute the vial of Ancef.

    A. What will be the concentration of this medication? _____

    B. What is Ancef's generic name? _____

    C. Is this an SVP or LVP? _____

    D. What size syringe and needle should be used to prepare this order?

    _____

4. Refer to the following pharmacy order. The concentration of the vancomycin stock bottle is 1 g/10 mL.

    A. How many milliliters of vancomycin are necessary for this order? _____

    | | | |
    |---|---|---|
    | TTC Pharmacy Lab | | |
    | Patient: Karen Snipe | ID#258490 | RM# 235 |
    | Prepared: 11:00 AM | Date: 09/18/03 | |
    | | | |
    | Rate: Over 60 min. | | |
    | Sodium Chloride  100 ml | | |
    | Vancomycin       500 mg | | |
    | | | |
    | Freq: q12h | | |
    | Exp. 9/21/03 | 11:00 AM | By: hds |

    B. What is the expiration date on this order? _____

    C. How many bags are necessary? _____

## Aseptic Technique

1. Turn on the flow hood 30 minutes before working in the hood.

2. Clean the work surface of the hood from back to front and the sides from top to bottom with 70% isopropyl alcohol and 4 × 4 gauze.

3. Assemble all supplies.

4. Calculate the amount required for each preparation.

5. Remove all jewelry and wash hands thoroughly.

6. Put on gown, hair cover, shoe cover, mask, and gloves.

Copyright © 2007 Elsevier, Inc. All rights reserved.

7. Working in the back of the hood, position supplies for preparation.

8. Sterilize (swab) all surfaces requiring needle entry.

9. Prepare all products needed.

10. Set aside prepared products for final check with the following:
    A. Bag or syringe prepared with label attached
    B. Drug vial used
    C. Syringe pulled back to amount added
    D. Filter needle if ampule used
    E. Initials on label
    F. IV seal on bag

11. Clean the hood before leaving the IV area.

Copyright © 2007 Elsevier, Inc. All rights reserved.

Give the abbreviations for the following terms.

1. Of each _____

2. Before meals _____

3. Right ear _____

4. Up to _____

5. As needed _____

6. Morning _____

7. Ampule _____

8. Amount _____

9. Left ear _____

10. As soon as possible _____

11. Around the clock _____

12. Both ears _____

13. Water _____

14. Twice a day _____

15. Blood pressure _____

16. Bowel movement _____

17. Body surface area _____

18. Centigrade _____

19. With _____

20. Cup _____

Copyright © 2007 Elsevier, Inc. All rights reserved.

Give the abbreviations for the following terms.

1. Complete blood count _____
2. Dram _____
3. Cubic centimeter _____
4. Deoxyribonucleic acid _____
5. Calcium _____
6. Dispense _____
7. Capsules _____
8. Chlorine _____
9. Discharge _____
10. Discontinue _____

11. Centimeter _____
12. Dilute _____
13. Complaint of _____
14. Drug Enforcement Administration _____
15. Central nervous system _____
16. Diagnosis _____
17. Compound _____
18. Day _____
19. Cerebrospinal fluid _____
20. Cesarean section _____

Copyright © 2007 Elsevier, Inc. All rights reserved.

Give the abbreviations for the following medical terms.

1. Alcohol _____

2. Electrocardiogram _____

3. Expired _____

4. Elixir _____

5. Fahrenheit _____

6. Grain _____

7. Iron _____

8. Gram _____

9. Fluid _____

10. Food and Drug Administration _____

11. Drops _____

12. Gastrointestinal _____

13. Hour _____

14. Water _____

15. At bedtime _____

16. Intravenous _____

17. Intrathecal _____

18. Intramuscular _____

19. Immune globulin G _____

20. History _____

Copyright © 2007 Elsevier, Inc. All rights reserved.

Give the abbreviations for the following medical terms.

1. Intravenous push _____

2. Kilocalorie _____

3. Kilogram _____

4. Potassium _____

5. Liter _____

6. Liquid _____

7. Microgram _____

8. As directed _____

9. Milliequivalent _____

10. Magnesium _____

11. Milligram _____

12. Minute _____

13. Mixture _____

14. Millimeter _____

15. Month _____

16. Magnetic resonance imaging _____

17. Sodium _____

18. Sodium chloride _____

19. Negative _____

20. Milliliter _____

Copyright © 2007 Elsevier, Inc. All rights reserved.

Give the abbreviations for the following medical terms.

1. Operating room _____
2. Ointment _____
3. Right eye _____
4. Nonsteroidal antiinflammatory drug _____
5. Nothing by mouth _____
6. In the night _____
7. Number _____
8. No known drug allergies _____
9. No known allergies _____
10. National formulary _____
11. Left eye _____
12. Over the counter _____
13. Each eye _____
14. Ounce _____
15. After meals _____
16. By _____
17. Afternoon _____
18. By mouth _____
19. Per rectum _____
20. Whenever necessary _____

Copyright © 2007 Elsevier, Inc. All rights reserved.

Give the abbreviations for the following medical terms.

1. Every _____

2. Every morning _____

3. Every day _____

4. Every hour _____

5. Four times a day _____

6. Every other day _____

7. Quantity sufficient _____

8. Quantity _____

9. Rule out _____

10. Prescription, recipe _____

11. Repeat _____

12. Without _____

13. Saturated _____

14. Shortness of breath _____

15. Solution _____

16. Subcutaneous _____

17. Label, let it be printed _____

18. One half _____

19. Sublingual _____

20. Dissolve _____

Copyright © 2007 Elsevier, Inc. All rights reserved.

Give the abbreviations for the following medical terms.

1. Urinary tract infection _____

2. United States Pharmacopeia _____

3. United States Adopted Names _____

4. Ointment _____

5. As directed _____

6. Teaspoonful _____

7. Triturate _____

8. Tincture _____

9. Three times a day _____

10. Temperature _____

11. Tablespoonful _____

12. Tablets _____

13. Sterile water for injection _____

14. Syringe, syrup _____

15. Suppository _____

16. Immediately _____

17. Vaginal _____

18. Volume _____

19. Verbal order _____

20. Vital signs _____

Copyright © 2007 Elsevier, Inc. All rights reserved.

Give the abbreviations for the following medical terms.

1. While awake _____
2. Times _____
3. Year _____
4. Oxygen _____
5. Potassium chloride _____
6. Angiotensin-converting enzyme _____
7. Aspirin _____
8. Acetaminophen _____
9. Penicillin _____
10. Tetracycline _____
11. Milk of magnesia _____
12. Morphine sulfate _____
13. Magnesium sulfate _____
14. Patient-controlled anesthesia _____
15. Hydrochloric acid _____
16. Carbon dioxide _____
17. Sodium bicarbonate _____
18. Zinc oxide _____
19. Calcium channel blocker _____
20. Phenobarbital _____

Copyright © 2007 Elsevier, Inc. All rights reserved.

ABBREVIATION QUIZ 9

Give the abbreviations for the following medical terms.

1. Hypertension _____
2. Myocardial infarction _____
3. Acquired immunodeficiency syndrome _____
4. Human immunodeficiency virus _____
5. Cancer _____

6. Gastroesophageal reflux disease _____
7. Congestive heart failure _____
8. Cerebrovascular accident _____
9. Deep vein thrombosis _____
10. Upper respiratory infection _____

Lab Sheets and Abbreviation Quizzes

Copyright © 2007 Elsevier, Inc. All rights reserved.

Give the acronyms for the following organizations.

1. Food and Drug Administration _____

2. Drug Enforcement Administration _____

3. American Society of Health-Systems Pharmacists _____

4. Pharmacy Technician Certification Board _____

5. American Pharmaceutical Association _____

6. National Association of the Boards of Pharmacy _____

7. Board of Pharmacy _____

8. Centers for Disease Control and Prevention _____

9. American Association for Pharmacy Technicians _____

10. Pharmacy Technician Education Council _____

11. Joint Commission on Accreditation of Healthcare Organizations _____

12. Health Care Financing Administration _____

13. Pharmacy and Therapeutics Committee _____

14. Drug Use Evaluation _____

15. Drug Utilization Review _____

Copyright © 2007 Elsevier, Inc. All rights reserved.